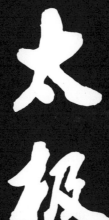

Tai Chi

TEN MINUTES TO HEALTH

Chia Siew Pang · Goh Ewe Hock

太极

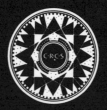

CRCS PUBLICATIONS
P.O. Box 1460
Sebastopol, CA 95473
USA

FIRST USA EDITION
INTERNATIONAL STANDARD BOOK NUMBER
0-916360-30-X

Library of Congress Cataloging-in-Publication Data

Chia, Siew Pang.
Tai chi : ten minutes to health.

Originally published: Taiji.   Singapore : Times
Books International, C 1983.
1. T'ai chi ch'üan.   I. Goh, Tommy Ewe Hock.
II. Title.
GV505.C467 1985   796.8'155   85-22388
ISBN 0-916360-30-X (pbk.)

Acknowledgements

The authors are grateful to a whole host of people who encouraged and assisted us in the production of this book. In particular, we are indebted to Fam, Danny and Soo Jin for putting in so much effort and providing cheerful and enthusiastic support.

Contents

Introduction

Tai chi, an ancient martial art based upon Taoist philosophy, probably developed in China during the Sung dynasty. It was initially taught and practised only in northern China. The Japanese invasion in the twentieth century stimulated its spread to other parts of the country while the communist takeover of the nation was largely responsible for its dissemination to Taiwan, Hong Kong and the countries of Southeast Asia. From these overseas centres the art was propagated even further.

Paradoxically, despite its popularity, there exists a good deal of misconception about tai chi. Some view it as a mild exercise. Yet those who practise other forms of martial art recognise it as a martial art that takes a long time to learn and even longer to perfect. Many will attest to its effectiveness, but just what makes it effective as a martial art no one seems to know.

This is not surprising. Relatively few people have mastered tai chi; fewer are willing to pass on knowledge of it. Most of those who do often describe only the basic tenets on which it is based, and even those in very vague and general terms. This is due, in part, to the Chinese (or perhaps Asian) tradition of reserving knowledge of the more intricate aspects of a martial art to those of proven loyalty and integrity. There are other factors that ensure a deep grounding of the art is passed on effectively to only a carefully selected handful. Few exponents, for example, would have sufficient motivation and self-discipline to ignore society's ever-persuasive attractions to undertake a prolonged period of painful practice and relative isolation essential for the mastery of the art. Respectability and a lucrative livelihood, the rewards a master of martial arts could look forward to in the past, are not such certain rewards in today's society.

What then is tai chi? How is it practised today? How does it differ from other martial art systems?

Its practice consists essentially of a series of continuous, slow, smooth and graceful moves executed with suppleness and in a relaxed manner. This practice, together with the maintenance of a straight and upright posture, form the bases of the art. These characteristics have led some people to describe tai chi as a 'soft' or 'internal' art. They recognise that its practice is diagrammatically opposed to the practice of the 'hard' or 'external' martial art systems exemplified by some of those taught in the Shaolin school. The 'external' or 'hard' schools emphasize forceful, rapid, staccato moves executed with strength and power. The more power, speed and accuracy the practitioner is able to concentrate in his move, the better he is judged to have executed it.

Is it conceivable that the practitioner of tai chi, a 'soft' art, would be able to withstand the devastating power of exponents of the 'hard' school? The fact is that a tai chi exponent is quite strong and very supple. His strength is concentrated in his legs and enables him to relax so as to leave his torso yielding and apparently 'soft'. Any force directed to the body would then be dissipated as there would be no solid surface to absorb its energy. The aggressor will find that he is unable to focus his attack and vent his power on a tai chi opponent, who escapes injury. Leg strength also enables the tai chi exponent to react like a coiled spring – recoiling away from a strong force and then springing back when that force is removed. The stronger the attacking force, the tighter the spring and the stronger the counter-attack.

How does the tai chi exponent develop such strength and suppleness? He does so through meticulous, consistent repetition of a predetermined set of moves of which, in this book, there are forty-four. The moves are made with the body relaxed and, when it is upright, completely straight. Relaxation promotes the transfer of body weight to the legs. The more you can relax, the greater the weight that sinks down to your legs. A straight posture permits the flow of *ji* (energy) and helps focus body weight onto a small area. A perfect combination of relaxation and a completely straight posture is difficult to attain as it frequently loads the leg muscles to an unbearable degree, causing pain – pain which often causes an exponent to either involuntarily tense up or to shift his position and lose the correct posture. This manoeuvre would lessen the load on the leg muscles and bring immediate relief, but it also reduces the value of the exercise to the practitioner. As in most endeavours, the benefit one derives in tai chi is directly proportional to the intensity of effort put in.

Why do we talk about an increased load on the legs? Aren't our legs carrying all our body weight all the time anyway? Consider what happens when you assume a hunched posture. Your body weight would be spread over a wider area than when you assume a straight, upright posture. If, for example, you weigh 70 kg and your weight is diffused over an area of 100 sq. cm, then the load that your legs carried would be 70/100 or 0.7 kg per sq. cm. The tai chi exponent who tries to focus his weight on a smaller area, say 50 sq. cm, would carry a load of 70/50 or 1.4 kg per sq. cm – twice as much weight! Continued exposure to an increased load permits the tai chi exponent to develop his leg muscles, particularly the thigh muscles, considerably. The increased leg strength not only gives the tai chi exponent explosive strength to push opponents 20–30 metres or more away but also blinding speed which enables him to move faster than his opponents.

In order to acquire such proficiency, an exponent must possess a great deal of patience and the spirit of perfectionism. Although tai chi exponents do practise regularly, from ignorance or laziness many do not follow the basic precepts meticulously. They inevitably adopt incorrect postures or tense up or do both, to reduce the load and thus ease the pain in their legs. Unless checked, a practitioner seldom progresses very far in the practice of the art. Yet correction cannot be done immediately. It has to be done gradually, a little during each session over a period of time, until the student's strength improves sufficiently to enable him to take on the increased loads that further correction will bring. It is relatively easy, therefore, to learn the moves of the tai chi exercise, but extremely difficult to master the art of tai chi. This is one of the main reasons why there are so few really good tai chi exponents today.

However, we do not attempt to produce expert tai chi exponents. We introduce the fundamentals of Yang tai chi (see 'Heritage' on pages 6–8), as taught by the late Cheng Mun-ch'ng, and hope that we can interest you sufficiently so that you will practise it as a basic form of exercise. Tai chi is a very good form of exercise, particularly for the older age groups. Despite its apparent effortlessness, a practitioner begins to perspire profusely after a few minutes of exercise – the amount seemingly disproportionate to the effort that appears to have been put in. Appearances, in the case of tai chi, are deceptive: we have recorded increases in pulse rate from a resting 70 per minute to 120 per minute after just 7 minutes of slow exercise.

It is best to study tai chi chuan from a teacher. It is vital, however, that the teacher understands and is willing to teach its fundamentals. Do not hesitate to query why a move should be made in a particular way, why a hand or a leg should be placed in just this position and not in another. The answer probably lies in the application of that move in a combat situation for, after all, tai chi is a potent martial art with its martial aspects often disguised by slow and apparently meaningless moves. It is beyond the scope of this book to go into these aspects. Do, however, ask someone why a particular posture is right and another wrong. You will find that once you have understood its meaning and use you will be better able to remember how the move should be performed.

The Heritage of Tai Chi

Tai chi came into prominence in the eighteenth century when Yang Lu-ch'an introduced it in Beijing. Prior to this, tai chi was reported to have been taught only to members of the Chen family living in a small village in Hopeh Province. Yang Lu-ch'an was the first non-member of the Chen family to be taught this most secret art. The following version of how this occurred was related by our teachers. We cannot vouch for its authenticity but nonetheless have recorded it as it gives an insight into and forms an interesting background for this ancient and rich art.

Yang Lu-ch'an was a pugilistic enthusiast. He studied the 'hard' schools of martial art from many tutors. One day, he had a heated discussion with a Chen and was beaten up for his pains. Yang was very frustrated as he realised his skill in martial art was very inferior to Chen's. He requested a return bout. During the interim he practised assiduously. In the return bout, he was again handled like a babe and thrashed so soundly by Chen that he forswore the practice of all other forms of martial art. He was determined to learn Chen's system.

He soon discovered that it was taught only to members of the Chen family and then only if the Chen stayed in a particular village – the Chen Chia Kou village. The Chen who defeated him was the nephew of the grandmaster. Yang wished to learn from the grandmaster but realised that a direct approach would be unsuccessful. He decided to 'steal' the art from the family. First he disguised himself as a beggar, then he made himself temporarily dumb by swallowing some hot charcoal. He hoped that the sight of a poor, suffering beggar outside his home would evoke the grandmaster's sympathy.

The ruse worked. Yang gained entry and was eventually employed as a servant in the grandmaster's household. He soon became a trusted servant and was given access to the inner courtyards of the family household. Here he spied on the Chen family as they practised. Religiously, he copied their moves and practised them in secret. He was able to benefit from this activity as he already had a good grounding in the martial art.

One night, as Yang was practising secretly, he suddenly found the grandmaster observing him. He was terrified. In those days in China, the price one paid for spying on other martial art systems was either one's head or right hand! The grandmaster, surprisingly, demanded neither. He merely said, 'Do you think I did not realise you were spying on us when we were practising? I allowed you to watch because I wanted to see how serious you were and how well you would benefit from the instruction. If you had shown neither interest nor skill, I would have killed you myself.'

On saying that, he tapped Yang three times on the head and walked away, leaving a puzzled but very relieved man. From that day, Yang went to the grandmaster's quarters every morning at 3 a.m. for personalised instruction in tai chi. During the day he did his chores as usual and no one in the family realised he was receiving secret instruction from the grandmaster.

One day the grandmaster explained why he had broken one of the strongest family traditions by teaching an outsider the secrets of the art. He had realised that by restricting the art to family members, tai chi would eventually decline in vitality. Family members would not have any incentive to practise well or to introduce new techniques since even those with less than perfect mastery of the art were far better than most practitioners from other schools of martial art. He reasoned that if he taught a talented and skilled outsider, like Yang, he would ensure that the essence of tai chi would not be lost to the world. Further, tai chi would remain a vigorous and vital art as not only would it be practised by many but also the family members would have to practise hard in order to avoid being beaten by their own art.

The tradition of selecting hardworking and dedicated students to pass on the knowledge of the art began with Yang and has persisted. Often masters would not accept payment from such students, whose only obligation was to learn the art well and, in turn, pass on their knowledge to other deserving students.

Thus Yang Lu-ch'an fulfilled his greatest desire and was personally instructed by the grandmaster for several long years. This grandmaster remained critical of the standard of the art practised by members of the family. At one of the annual competitions held among members of the Chen family, he noted that none of the younger members was able to defeat an old man like himself. It was pointed out that this was because he had so much more experience and practice. Since the proficiency of an exponent was related to the amount of practice and as age did not impair one's ability in the art, they were confident that when they reached his age they would equal or better his skill.

Then the grandmaster dropped his bombshell: 'If I can produce someone younger than myself, who has acquired sufficient skill through thoughtful and diligent practice, to defeat all of you, what would you all have to say then?'

This statement was received with much laughter. The grandmaster's claim was treated with some derision when the family discovered that this superman was none other than their servant, Yang Lu-ch'an. Laughter turned to disbelief as, one after another, members of the Chen family were beaten by Yang. Gradually, their feelings hardened into anger as they realised that not only had their grandmaster trained an outsider, he had done it so well that he could defeat all members of the family. They felt cheated and betrayed.

'Yang Lu-ch'an will go forth and teach the world tai chi. If you all do not practise well enough, you will soon find that others will be better than you in your own art. Although I have broken our family tradition by teaching an outsider, I have ensured that the knowledge of the art will not die but will blossom and develop over the years.'

With those words, the grandmaster personally escorted Yang out of the village and gave him his blessings to spread the knowledge of tai chi. Yang lost no time in fulfilling his teacher's wishes. He had to establish tai chi as an effective martial art system before he could attract any good students to his school. In order to do this, he wandered all over Hopeh Province, taking on all challengers. In his first year he carried a flag that proclaimed he was the best martial art exponent and challenged anyone who disputed this claim. The flag was displayed in taverns, marketplaces and other public places. It soon attracted many challengers for all serious martial art practitioners are proud of displaying their skill. Furthermore, a proven martial art exponent in those days could earn an honourable and comfortable living by providing escort service for the richer merchants and travellers or by teaching his art.

Yang Lu-ch'an was never defeated in any of his bouts. He continued in his travels for a total of three years. His flag, by this time, recorded all his past victories and he called himself the 'Unbeatable Yang'. He also claimed that he practised the martial art system, tai chi chuan – 'grand ultimate fist'. Despite all these claims, the number of challengers dropped. So Yang went to Beijing and started a school of tai chi. Here he teamed up with two other 'soft' or 'internal' martial art schools (Hsing I and Pa Kua) and together they challenged, defeated and expelled all other martial art schools from Beijing. For a very long time afterwards, only these three schools of martial art were taught in Beijing.

Following Yang's death, his version of tai chi, now known as Yang tai chi, was taught mainly by members of his family. His grandson, Yang Cheng-fu, formalised the teaching of tai chi into a set of 81 moves which took a student some time to learn and about 15–20 minutes to complete. One of his better students, Cheng Mun-ch'ng, updated this version by weeding out the more repetitive and impractical moves. He retained the essence of the art by neither introducing any new moves nor attempting to change Yang Cheng-fu's interpretation of the art. Thus the basics of Yang tai chi as taught by the originator Yang Lu-ch'an were preserved, and today, this version of tai chi is the one which most closely resembles the original form. It is this version which was taught to Chia Siew Pang by Cheng Mun-ch'ng and which is presented in this manual.

We have described briefly the evolution and development of one of the more popular forms of tai chi. This version has stood the test of time. Today, it is still widely practised in many parts of the world. However, it is not the only version of tai chi that has developed over the years. In attempts to improve upon what they have learnt, several have introduced their interpretations of the art; the result has been the development of many schools of tai chi. Among the better known versions are Chen tai chi, Wu tai chi and Sun tai chi. Many later versions introduced modifications to the original system. Sun tai chi, for example, incorporates some of the techniques of other 'soft' martial art systems. All this reflects the rich heritage and versatility of the ancient art.

Tai Chi for Health

The majority of those who practise tai chi do so mainly for the benefits it gives as an exercise. Relatively few learn it only for its martial aspects. As an exercise, tai chi is suitable for people of all ages, particularly those on the wrong side of thirty. The very nature of the art stimulates blood circulation, loosens and limbers up joints and at the same time promotes mental relaxation.

It has been claimed that tai chi, when practised diligently, will help and even cure certain morbid conditions. Some have reported that the practice of tai chi can produce remissions for organic diseases like tuberculosis and diabetes mellitus, but do not offer any rational explanation as to how this is achieved. Although tai chi would undoubtedly promote health, the more extravagant claims of its therapeutic benefits should be viewed in their correct perspective. These claims should be based upon carefully planned and executed studies and not solely upon the observation of isolated cases.

How would tai chi compare with other forms of exercise? One unique feature is that it promotes mental relaxation. In this it is like yoga and has been described as 'meditation in motion'. In practising tai chi the exponent never gets heated up over 'missing that damn putt' or losing a game. He is calm and relaxed with all tensions of the day eased away.

Tai chi exercises the cardio-pulmonary system, particularly when it is correctly practised. A half-hour tai chi workout would be equivalent to the exercise benefit derived from a three-hour game of golf. It is, however, a less intensive exercise than either squash or tennis.

One great advantage that tai chi has as an exercise is its convenience. Only ten minutes' exercise is all that is required for a practice session. It certainly beats rearranging schedules to fit in a round of golf or even a jogging session! What is more, tai chi can be practised in a relatively small area, with no special equipment or companion. Your office, bedroom, lounge, patio, garden – just about any open space 15 metres square can be used for the practice of tai chi. It can, therefore, be practised in your own home, at practically any time, with minimal expense and by yourself. Most important, you will always feel good, relaxed, refreshed and invigorated after a tai chi session.

As in other exercises, do not practise tai chi when you suffer an acute illness like influenza or diarrhoea. It is much better and certainly safer to resume practice after your recovery. Although you do not require any special equipment, you should always use a pair of flat-soled shoes during practice to avoid injury to your soles. A soft, loose, sweat-absorbing shirt and loose, baggy pants will be an asset as they permit free movement. Avoid using skin-tight pants and shirts during practice – these not only hamper blood circulation, they also cause some discomfort. For the same reasons, tight-fitting rings should be taken off before practice.

The beauty of practising tai chi is that, apart from getting considerable physical exercise, you are learning, quite by accident perhaps, an ancient martial art. Unconsciously you will imbibe its principles and when this occurs, you will inherit some of the values and qualities the Chinese prize highly – patience, perseverance, tolerance, discipline and confidence.

The Tai Chi Exercise

The tai chi exercise consists of an interlinked series of 44 moves (37 of them different) that should take 7–8 minutes to complete.

This exercise is taught in four chapters, demarking areas that a beginner should first become familiar with before proceeding further. This is the first time that such a detailed step-by-step instruction of this art has been presented. It will guide the student in his practice as it not only shows how he can proceed from one move to another, but also breaks down each move into its component parts. As we feel it would be difficult to follow the instructions from the text alone, a carefully phased sequence of photographs and diagrams have been used to simplify the exercise. The student will be able to see exactly where to place his feet, and what to do with his body and his hands in the meantime. Chia will demonstrate what he has learnt from Cheng Mun-ch'ng and how he himself has taught over the last 30 years.

Presentation

In order to follow the instructions given, it is essential that you understand how the material is being presented. Basically, each move, or a particular segment of it, is presented on one page.

The name of the move is set out above brief explanatory notes which highlight points you should keep in mind while executing the move. Many of the basic principles to be borne in mind will not be repeated *ad nauseum* and you should refer regularly to a summary of these in your practice (see Rapid Reminders on page 12).

Next to the text, in two rows of photographs, the move is broken down into its component parts, illustrating how one part of the move is linked with the next. The photographs in the top row show Chia carrying out these component movements facing you while the corresponding photographs in the second row show exactly the same movements, this time viewed from the back. Care has been taken to minimise distortion by ensuring that the photographs are taken from about the same angle and distance.

A row of diagrams follow the photographs. These show the correct positioning of feet and distribution of weight between the feet as the moves are executed. Brief notes in the diagrams indicate the direction you should face (FRONT) and the angle and direction in which you need to turn your body.

Names of moves have been retained in their original *hanyu pinyin*. The literal English translation of these names have been included, though we have reservations about their use: without a correct understanding of the cultural background and the innuendos of the Chinese language, an English translation of names of tai chi moves may result in a loss of their beauty. Their inclusion in this book, however, may aid those for whom Chinese names are difficult to remember.

Terminology

One of the underlying precepts of tai chi is the ability to minimise tension in the upper parts of your body. To achieve this, movement in any one limb is restricted to only one joint at a time. Thus a precise knowledge of the joints involved in a movement is essential. The description included in this text can prove difficult to comprehend unless some explicit terminology is used to describe the moves. In order to minimise confusion, a short explanation and illustrations of the terms used are presented here.

ABDUCTION/ADDUCTION These refer to movements at the major ball-and-socket joints at the shoulders and hips.

ABDUCTION This refers to raising the upper arm or thigh, i.e. moving the upper part of a limb away from the body.

ADDUCTION This refers to bringing a limb toward the body. It produces a movement which is the exact reverse of abduction.

The motion resulting from either abduction or adduction can take place in two planes:

1 Forward or backward, i.e. anteriorly or posteriorly, and

2 Sideways, i.e. laterally.

In this text we have restricted the use of abduction/adduction to movements of upper arms and thighs.

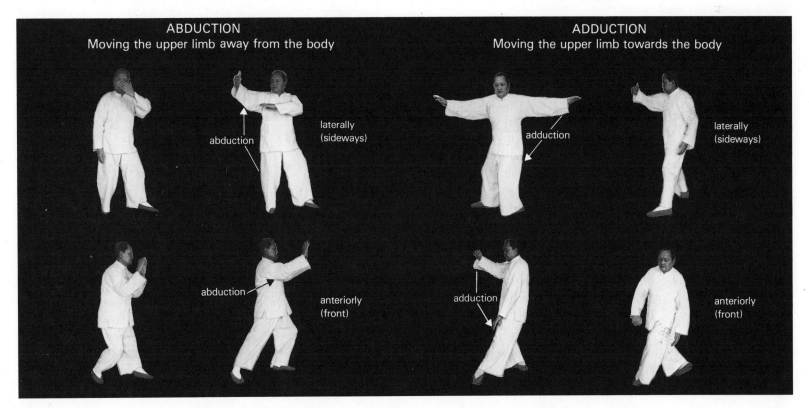

ABDUCTION
Moving the upper limb away from the body

abduction

laterally (sideways)

abduction

anteriorly (front)

ADDUCTION
Moving the upper limb towards the body

adduction

laterally (sideways)

adduction

adduction

anteriorly (front)

FLEXION/ EXTENSION	These refer to the movements that take place in the hinge joints in the limbs, i.e. the elbow, wrist, knee and ankle joints.
FLEXION	Flexion refers to the bending of the joint to bring the upper and lower parts of a limb toward each other.
EXTENSION	This refers to the reverse action which results in the two parts of a limb moving away from each other.

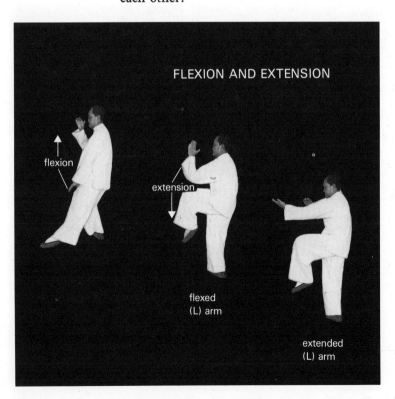

FLEXION AND EXTENSION

flexion

extension

flexed
(L) arm

extended
(L) arm

Rapid Reminders

A few basic concepts should constantly be borne in mind. It would be useful to read these carefully both before you begin your exercise and upon its completion. You will find that your appreciation of the points raised will have changed. You may also discover after practising for a while that you have forgotten some of the basic precepts. Reading the points below regularly will aid you in your practice of tai chi.

SLOWNESS	Try to execute all movements as slowly as you can. Concentrate on the move you are carrying out to get it as precise as possible. Try and visualise the resulting moves and the joints which are involved in producing them. Do not rush through the exercise as it will not benefit you in the long run.
CONTINUITY	All moves should flow continuously and without pause, from one to the other. Avoid pausing to adjust the positioning of limbs and body. This, though essential, should not be carried out in the midst of an exercise.
PRECISION	It will not be possible to achieve the correct posture easily or early during your practice. Initially, what is important is your understanding of the correct postures and the basis on which these are achieved. Continue attempting, each time you practise, to attain the correct postures. You will find these can only be achieved when you have developed sufficient strength.

RELAXATION
Your body and upper limbs should, at all times, be as relaxed as possible. Your shoulders and chest should never be tense. To achieve this your leg muscles, particularly the thigh muscles, will be placed under stress and will ache after each session.

WEIGHT DISTRIBUTION
Body weight should never be equally distributed on both legs for any length of time, except at the very beginning and end of the exercise. Your weight should be channelled through one point, as far as possible, to the ground. Occasionally you will see diagrams showing positions where the weight is equally distributed on both feet. These are transient positions and the diagrams merely illustrate the transfer of weight from one foot to another. When one foot, in a particular position, bears only a fraction of your weight and immediately afterwards carries the brunt of your weight, there must be a point where it carries 50 per cent of your weight: this is what the diagram illustrates. Remember, however, that it is not a desirable position and you should avoid keeping the weight of your body evenly distributed over any prolonged period.

BREATHING
Always breathe in naturally through your nose and out through your mouth. Do not expel breath forcibly from your lungs or combine exotic breathing techniques with the exercise, particularly during the early stages.

EQUIPMENT
Do wear a pair of flat-soled shoes during practice. High-heeled shoes and bare feet should be avoided as you will be exerting a great deal of pressure on your feet during the exercise. Loose clothing, particularly of cotton, is recommended. When you practise outdoors, especially in the evenings, it is advisable to wear clothing which will cover elbows and knees.

PRACTICE
Many teachers hold the view that the effort put into morning practice results in 2–3 times greater benefit than a similar effort in the evening. Whatever time you find convenient, it is generally better to practise consistently at set times daily than to randomise your practice time. Regularity and consistency of practice is more beneficial than intense, short periods of enthusiastic practice. When you have learnt the entire sequence of moves and are proficient, you may wish to carry out three sets of the entire exercise daily with 3–5 minutes' rest between sets. This would help to improve your practice of the art in the shortest time possible.

POSTURE
Stationary While stationary and upright, you should always hold your body straight. This can be achieved if you keep your:
- head up and eyes focused on your outstretched hand and not on your feet,
- chin tucked in comfortably,

- chest relaxed,
- abdomen taut and pulled in,
- coccyx pulled in and upward.

In motion While moving from one position to another, try to maintain an even, level height throughout. Avoid bobbing up and down. This can be achieved if you keep your knees slightly flexed as you move and shift your weight from one foot to another. Keeping your height on an even plane will increase the strain on your leg muscles and channel the force generated downward.

Hips At the completion of a move, the hips should be pulled in until the line linking both hips is at right angles to your front foot.

LIMBS

Lower limbs
- Never move more than one joint in a limb simultaneously.
- Always place feet firmly on the ground before you move either forward or backward. Avoid moving *and* planting a foot down at the same time.
- Your front foot should always point in the direction you are facing or going to face at the completion of that move.
- Always turn your feet through 45° or multiples of 45°. The angle described by the heels of your feet should also be 45° or multiples of 45°.

Knees
- Knees should always be kept slightly bent (flexed) at the end of a move. In the text you will be instructed to 'straighten your leg'. This is important as it not only enables you to shift your weight easily from one foot to another but also to generate the force which is necessary to attack an opponent. However, *do not straighten your leg completely;* always keep a reserve by maintaining your knee slightly flexed.
- The bent knees should point in the direction of their respective toes.
- Never extend your knees beyond the level of your toes.

Upper limbs
- Only move one joint in either limb at any one time.
- Avoid exerting any force or tension in your forearms.
- Whenever you punch out with a clenched fist, never rotate your wrist at the end of the move. Keep your wrist firm with your knuckles perpendicular and *not* parallel to the ground.
- Whenever your palms are open, keep your fingers extended and separated from each other. If you have maintained the correct posture, your fingers will begin to tingle after a little while.

The Training Programme

It is always helpful to work out a programme or schedule that you know you can adhere to. This set target will act as a measure of your achievements.

A reasonable target to set yourself to learn this sequence of 44 moves may be 40 weeks. This assumes that you will:
- practise daily, and
- learn one new move every week.

If you have ever learnt tai chi or any other martial art or participated regularly in some active game, you would probably be able to achieve results in a shorter period. For the average person learning tai chi the very first time, thirty minutes to one hour should be spent during each session in this 40-week period.

While learning each new move it is essential that its component parts be analysed and thoroughly understood. You may find that, with time, you tend to forget the fundamentals of the moves. When this happens, you will progressively adopt bad habits. At this stage, it is important to spend time reviewing the basic components of the moves. With this knowledge you will be able to begin correcting yourself. One way to do this is to run through a mental checklist for each different move.

Prior to learning any move, learn and master the relaxation exercise. Then, during your daily practice session, carry out the relaxation exercise at least ten times – five turns to each side. After this, analyse the new move in detail, running through all the different stages shown in this book. Repeat the new move a minimum of ten times to commit it to memory. Finally incorporate this with the other moves learnt previously and repeat the entire sequence up to the new move a minimum of five times.

CHECKLIST

WEIGHT	• distribution/'loading' on feet.
HEIGHT	• level height, particularly during the shift of weight from one foot to another.
POSTURE	• straight, upright posture achieved by: coccyx pulled in and upward, stomach pulled inward, chest and shoulders relaxed, chin tucked in, eyes focused on outstretched hand.
MOVEMENT	• slow, continuous and relaxed. Flow from one position to another and merge imperceptibly. • mind concentrating only on moves that are being carried out. Avoid thinking of other things. • synchronisation of leg, body, hand and head movements.
LIMBS	**Feet** • toe direction, • angle between heels, • spacing between feet. **Hands** • direction of palms, • direction of knuckles in a clenched fist, • spread and extended fingers in an open hand, • relaxed forearms, • flexed elbows.

Relaxation Exercise

Like any other exercise, it is advisable not to start your practice of tai chi 'cold'. You will benefit more from practice if you do some preliminary exercises to loosen your joints and to stimulate your muscles. There are several loosening or relaxation exercises to choose from. One of the more comprehensive ones is illustrated here for your practice.

First assume a stance similar to that described for Fig. 1 *(yù bèi shì)*. The **feet** should be placed apart with about shoulder width distance between them. Keep **knees** slightly bent and pointing outward. Pull your **coccyx** in and upward and, at the same time, hold your **stomach** in. Relax both **chest** and **shoulders.** Pull in your **chin** and keep **eyes** focused on some distant object in front of you. While in this position, keep weight equally distributed on both feet.

Rotate **wrists** so both palms face forward and extend fingers to separate them. Abduct both **shoulders** laterally and raise both arms above you with palms facing forward (Fig. A). Now shift 90 per cent of your weight onto the **(L) foot**. Adduct both **shoulders** to bring arms to your side. Then, *and only then,* flex both **elbows** to raise the forearms. Coordinate this with a 90° turn to your right, pulling in your (R) hip for that extra bit of torsion that will bring your hips in line with your shoulders. This turn together with the flexion of the elbows will bring your (L) arm in front

and the (R) arm behind you. Let both arms fall naturally and avoid putting any force into the swing. If you had done this right, the arms would first fall vertically and then be pulled across the body and upward. The arms would then flow with the force of gravity. If your shoulders had been relaxed, the (L) hand would reach the (R) shoulder. The (R) hand would be behind you with (R) palm facing away from you. As you turn, pivot on your (R) heel and turn **(R) foot** 90° to the right. This will bring you to face the direction your front foot is pointing (Fig. B).

Now extend both **elbows** to allow the forearms to fall by your side. Synchronise this with a 90° turn, by both **body** and **(R) foot,** to your left. While doing this shift some of your weight back to your **(R) foot** so that it carries about half your weight. When this is done rotate wrists and adduct **shoulders** to raise both arms above you (Fig. C). You will now have returned to the posture with which you began this exercise.

Repeat the same sequence of moves, this time turning to your left. Your weight should now be on your (R) and not your (L) foot and it is the (R) and not the (L) arm that is now in front of you. When you have returned to the starting position of the exercise you would have completed one sequence of this relaxation exercise.

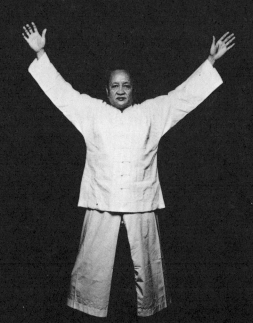

FIG. A

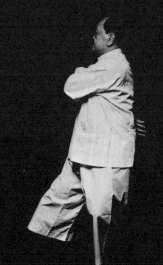

FIG. B

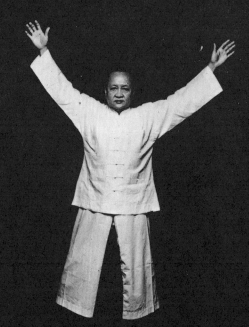

FIG. C

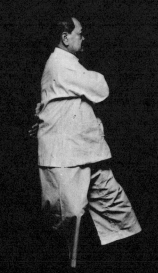

FIG. D

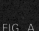

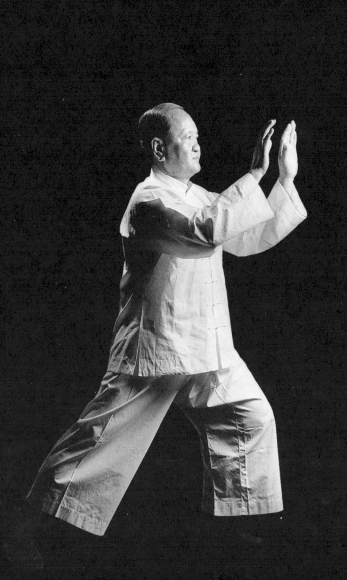

Chapter One

The first chapter of this exercise consists of thirteen moves. Although there are relatively few moves to master, you will probably find this one of the harder chapters. There are several reasons for this.

It may be the first time you will be required to consciously coordinate and synchronise movements of your head, hands and feet. If you have never participated in any active game, you will find this – initially at least – a major task. Like everything else, with practice you will gradually discover it becomes less of a chore and your hands and feet will no longer move awkwardly as you learn just where to put them.

There is also the problem of remembering the sequence of moves. Initially, when you are taught only a few moves, it will be difficult to practise regularly, largely because there are insufficient moves to stimulate your interest. When you learn more moves, you will find your practice is often interrupted because you forget just how one move is linked to another. It seems to

you this never occurs when you practise with your instructor. *Then* the moves and their sequence seem so easy, so logical, until you are by yourself . . . and that one move, the link, is totally beyond recall. It is therefore useful to have a practical manual on tai chi even when you have an instructor to teach you the art. The manual will serve as a useful reference when you practise by yourself.

Minimise your problems by limiting your study. Do not try to learn more than one move per session – certainly not more than two a week. Do, however, remember to ask – in detail – how the move should be carried out and then try to attain it during your practice session. You will find this helps you understand the principles and intricacies of each move much better. Remember that regular, constant practice is essential for mastery of tai chi. The person who puts in tremendous effort in periodic bursts of enthusiasm will eventually find himself lagging behind the patient plodder who does a bit each day, but does that little bit every day.

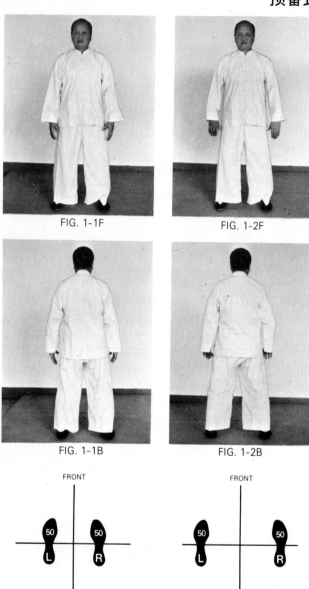

FIG. 1-1F　　　　　FIG. 1-2F

FIG. 1-1B　　　　　FIG. 1-2B

Keep weight evenly distributed on both feet.

Yù bèi shì

Preparation

This preparatory movement precedes every exercise. Stand with **feet** together. Move them apart until the distance between them is equal to the width of your shoulders. Body weight should be equally distributed on **both feet** and soles kept flat on the ground. Bend **knees** slightly. They should not extend beyond the toes. Turn kneecaps outward till they point toward the toes.

Keep your **spine** straight, pulling coccyx upward and inward. Hold **head** erect and look straight ahead with chin tucked comfortably in. If your head is bent either forward or backward, you will find the weight on your soles focused either toward the toes or heel.

Relax **shoulders** and pull them slightly down and rotate them outward so they become slightly rounded. Allow **arms** to hang loosely by your sides and hold them slightly away from the body and bent at the **elbows.** Your palms should initially face inward (Fig. 1–1). Later rotate wrists so that backs of hands face forward (Fig. 1–2).

Check that the different parts of your body are relaxed, paying particular attention to chest and stomach. When you are able to attain this position correctly, you will find that the tips of your fingers will tingle as blood circulation through them is enhanced.

Tài jí qǐ shì

Beginning

The second movement can be divided into six separate parts. The first three involve only the hands with position and weight distribution on legs remaining unchanged.

First abduct **shoulders** to raise both arms in front of you till they are at shoulder level. **Wrists** should be relaxed and hands held at an angle of about 45° to the arms. Keep **fingers** separate from each other and do not curl them up to form a fist. Note that Chia raises both arms in front and not at an acute angle to the body (Fig. 2-1). Rotating both shoulders forward at the end of the first movement will help achieve this.

At this point, flex both **elbows** and raise forearms to an upright position (Fig. 2-2). Continue the move by extending and straightening **wrists** so palms open forward. Extend **fingers** so they are straightened and held apart from each other (Fig. 2-3). Notice that in this sequence you have moved only the joints of your arm, starting with the largest (shoulder joints) and ending with the smallest (finger joints).

Do not stop but follow through the move by adducting **shoulders** then extending **elbows** in order to bring arms by your side. Rotate **shoulders** so that your arms will be held slightly away from your body with backs of palms facing forward. Note that you are now back in exactly the same posture held at the end of the first movement (Fig. 1-2) and that, throughout this movement, you have moved only one joint at a time.

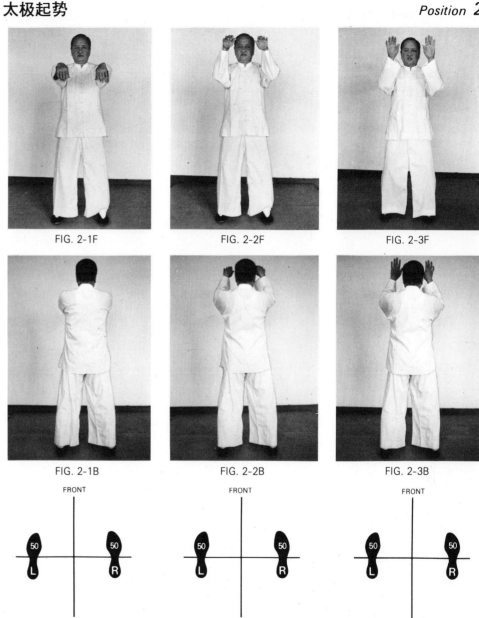

FIG. 2-1F   FIG. 2-2F   FIG. 2-3F

FIG. 2-1B   FIG. 2-2B   FIG. 2-3B

Keep weight evenly distributed on both feet.

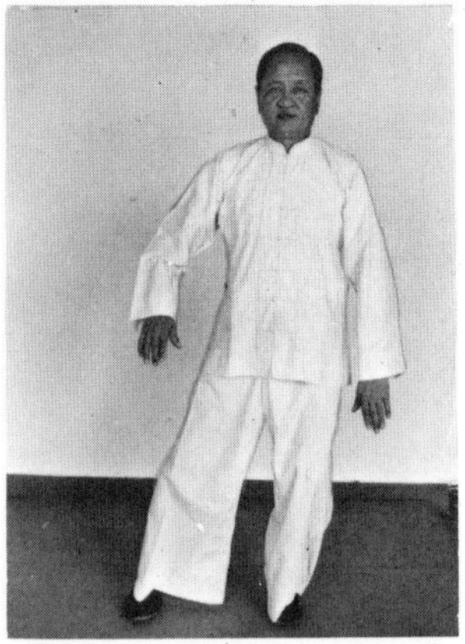

太极起势

FIG. 2-4F

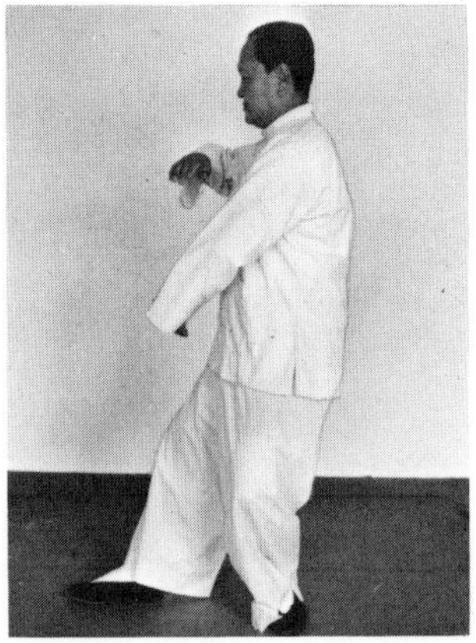

FIG. 2-5F

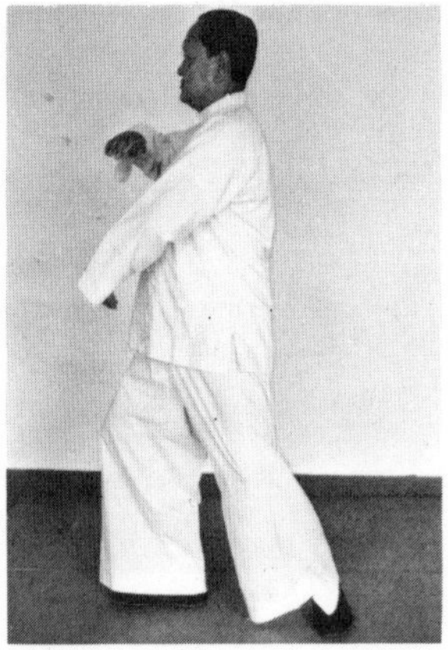

FIG. 2-6F

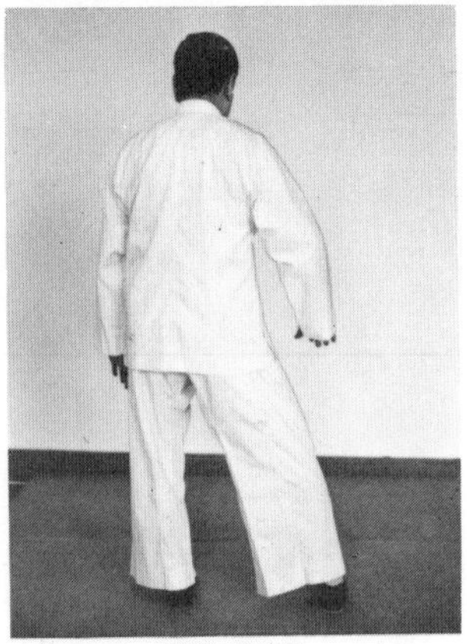

FIG. 2-4B

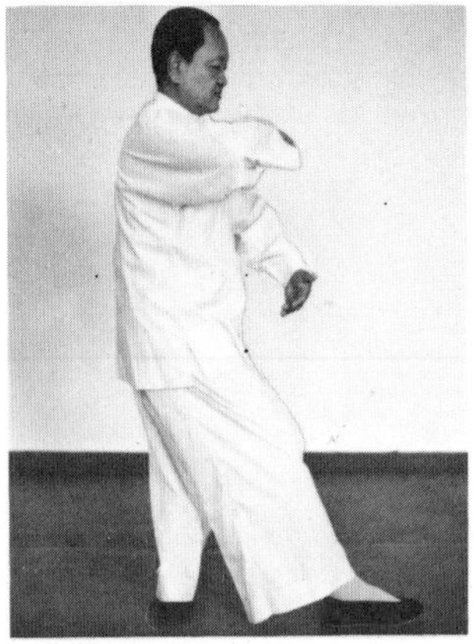

FIG. 2-5B

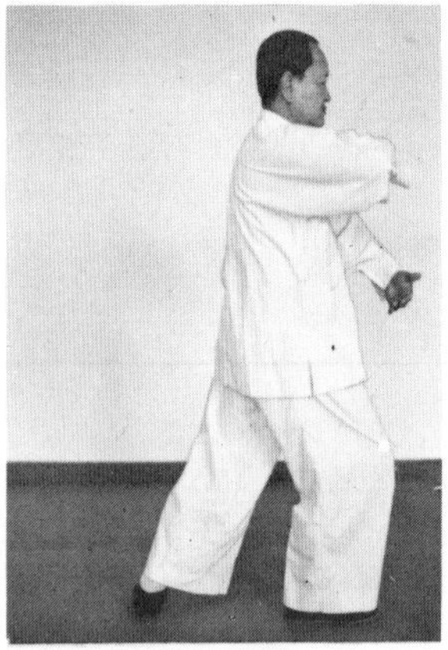

FIG. 2-6F

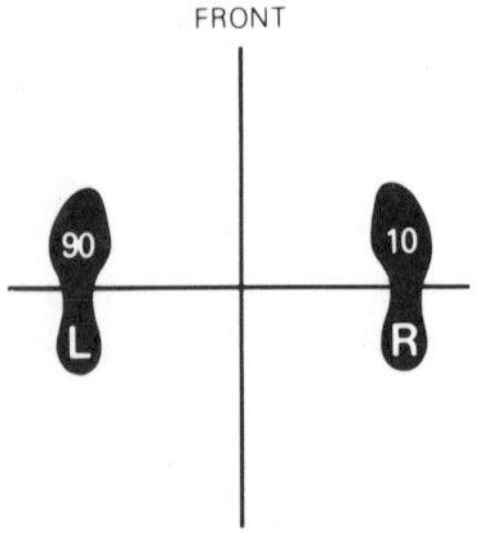

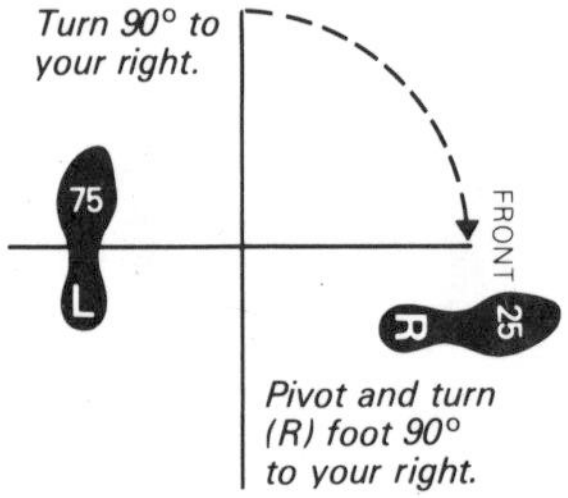

FRONT

90   10
L   R

Turn 90° to
your right.

75   FRONT
L   25
     R

Pivot and turn
(R) foot 90°
to your right.

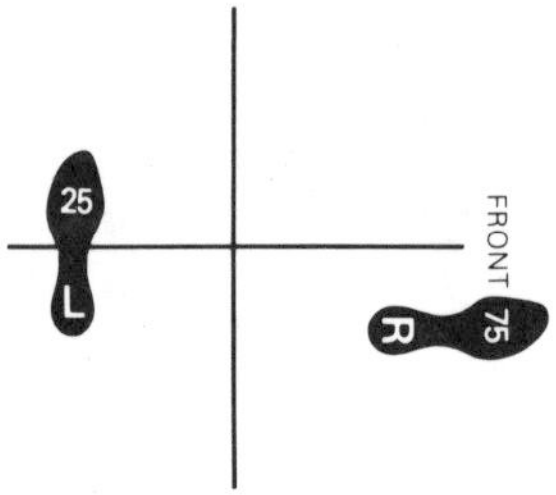

25   FRONT
L   75
     R

Initially move to your left, then turn 90° and move forward on front (R) foot.

Tài jí qǐ shì
Beginning

Now, to end the second movement. Relax **(L) hip** and move to your left so most of your weight is supported only by **(L) foot.** At the same time abduct **(R) shoulder** and raise (R) upper arm (Fig. 2-4). Rotate **shoulder** to raise (R) forearm till it is in line with upper arm and both are parallel to the floor (Fig. 2-5).

Next, pivot on (R) heel and **turn** 90° to the **right.** Your **(R) foot** should turn with your body. This will position both feet in such a manner that not only will they form a 90° angle between them but also both heels will be in line with each other.

When you have completed your turn your (R) arm should still be in front of you with the **palm** facing downward. Rotate **(L) wrist** so (L) palm faces upward, then flex **(L) elbow** to draw (L) forearm across the body until both **palms** face each other. At this stage, most of your weight should still be concentrated on the **(L) leg** (Fig. 2-5).

Finally, move forward, transferring at least 75 per cent of your weight to the front **(R) foot.** In your forward movement, ensure that you maintain the same height throughout and check that the **(R) knee** does not extend beyond the toes (Fig. 2-6). This completes the second movement.

Zuǒ péng shǒu

Ward off, left

The third move begins with your shifting more weight onto the **(R) foot.** When this is completed, lift **(L) foot** and move it straight ahead. Place heel where toes were (Fig. 3–1). Synchronise this movement with a 45° **turn** to your left. Do not move your hands at this stage. Most of your weight should still be on your (R) foot throughout.

The next part consists essentially of shifting weight from (R) to (L) foot. This is best described in two parts. First straighten **(R) leg.** Coordinate this with the movements of your arms. Adduct **(R) shoulder** and extend **(R) elbow** to allow (R) arm to sink to your side. At the same time abduct **(L) shoulder** to raise (L) upper arm until it is parallel to the ground. When it is in position, keep (L) elbow slightly flexed, so (L) forearm is in line with and at right angles to the upper arm. Note that your (L) palm faces the centre of your body. At this point your weight should be about equally distributed on both feet (Fig. 3–2).

Complete the 90° turn by turning another 45° to your left, keeping your hands still in relation to your body. Head movements should be coordinated with the rest of the body. You can achieve this if you remember to keep your eyes focused on your (L) palm all the time. Simultaneously, keeping the (R) heel stationary, your back **(R) foot** should also turn 45° to the left. At the end of the move, pull in your **hips** to ensure that they are in line with your shoulders. At this point most of your weight (about 75 per cent) should be on your front (L) foot (Fig. 3–3).

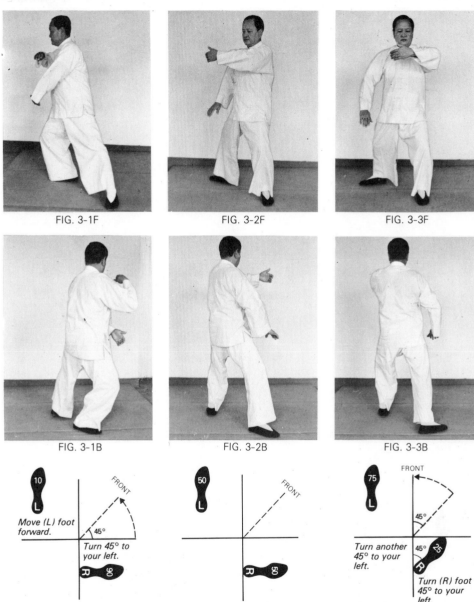

FIG. 3-1F   FIG. 3-2F   FIG. 3-3F

FIG. 3-1B   FIG. 3-2B   FIG. 3-3B

Shift weight to front (L) foot.

揽雀尾（棚手）

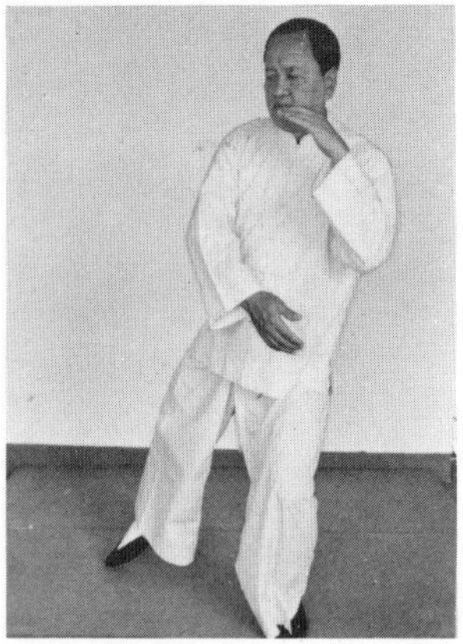

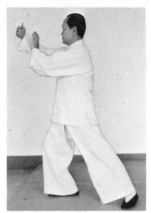

FIG. 4-1F

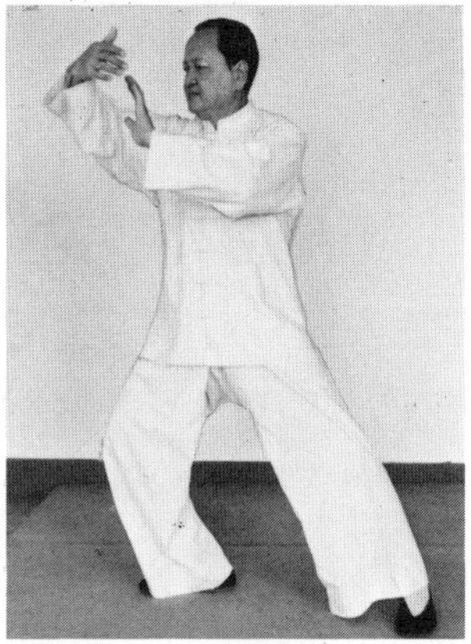

FIG. 4-2F

FIG. 4-3F

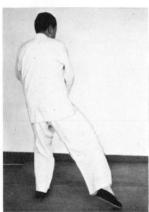

FIG. 4-1B

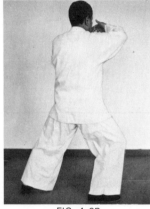

FIG. 4-2B

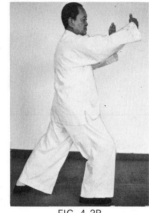

FIG. 4-3B

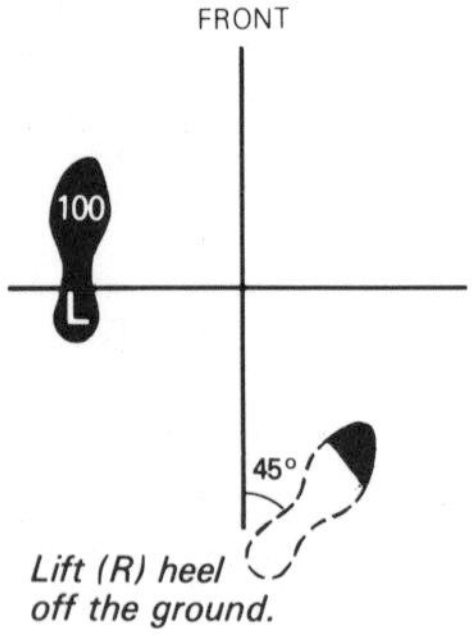

FRONT

100
L

45°

Lift (R) heel
off the ground.

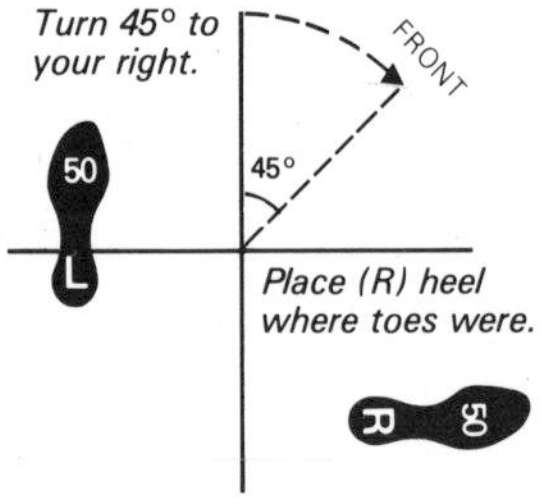

Turn 45° to
your right.

FRONT

50
L

45°

Place (R) heel
where toes were.

R 50

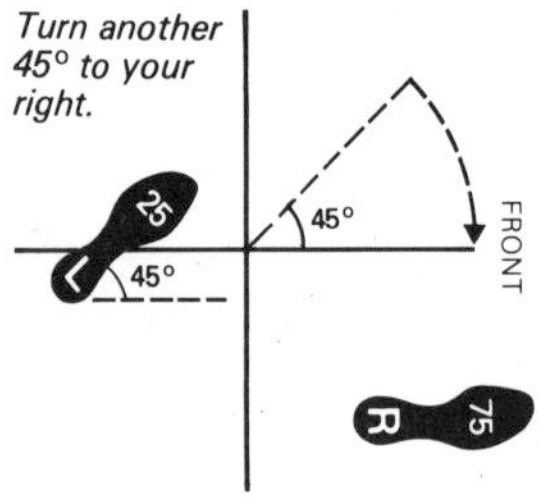

Turn another
45° to your
right.

FRONT

25
L

45°

45°

R 75

Shift weight to front (R) foot.

Lǎn què wěi (péng shǒu)

Grasp sparrow's tail, ward off

This is a composite of four different moves – *péng, lí, jǐ* and *àn*. These are frequently used and hence important moves to master in tai chi.

Péng shǒu forms the first part. It can be described in three parts. First shift weight onto the front **(L) foot** by lifting the **(R) heel**. In this position, adduct **(L) shoulder** to permit (L) elbow to move toward you and sink to your side with (L) forearm remaining upright. Your **(L) palm** is facing forward. Next rotate **(R) wrist** and turn (R) palm till it faces upward. Then, keeping (R) elbow slightly flexed, adduct **(R) shoulder** to pull (R) arm across the body from right to left (Fig. 4–1).

Now move **(R) foot** straight ahead and place (R) heel where (R) toes were. Turn body 45° to your right. Gradually shift weight to **(R) foot** by straightening (L) leg. (Do not straighten the (L) leg completely but keep it slightly bent with the knee facing the toes.) As you do this, abduct **(R) shoulder** till (R) upper arm is in line with shoulder. Rotate (R) shoulder to lift (R) forearm to eye level. Both palms should now face each other and you can imagine you are holding a ball between them (Fig. 4–2).

Turn **body** another 45° to your right. As you execute this, pull in (R) hip, keeping height constant. The back **(L) foot** should also turn 45° in conjunction with your body and it should carry only a small proportion of your weight at this point. Keep **(L) knee** bent and sole flat on the ground (Fig. 4–3). Remember that this turn is made essentially by your body and not with your hands.

Lǎn què wěi (lí shǒu)

Grasp sparrow's tail, roll back

Lí shǒu, the second part of the movement, can be divided in two. First relax **(R) hip** and move backward, keeping body straight so that the back **(L) foot** now carries most of your weight. While doing so, turn **(L) wrist** so (L) palm faces your body and then flex **(L) elbow** so the (L) forearm is pulled toward your body. This should be continued till (L) forearm is parallel to the floor and **(L) hand** is below (R) elbow. At the same time, rotate **(R) shoulder** to let (R) elbow sink downward with (R) forearm now assuming an upright position (Fig. 4–4).

The next part of the move is relatively simple and consists of focusing nearly all your weight on the back (L) leg while you turn slightly to your left. First begin turning 45° to your left, relax and allow all your weight to sink to your feet. Adduct **(L) shoulder** and extend **elbow** so **(L) arm** falls to your side. Also adduct **(R) shoulder** to pull (R) elbow in and downward toward you. Then as you turn to your left, rotate **(R) shoulder** to cause (R) forearm to fall toward your left till it is parallel to your body. In this way the (R) forearm will sweep across your body and end with the (R) hand pointing toward the (L) knee. Try to keep your front **(R) foot** flat on the ground as you carry out this part of the move (Fig. 4–5).

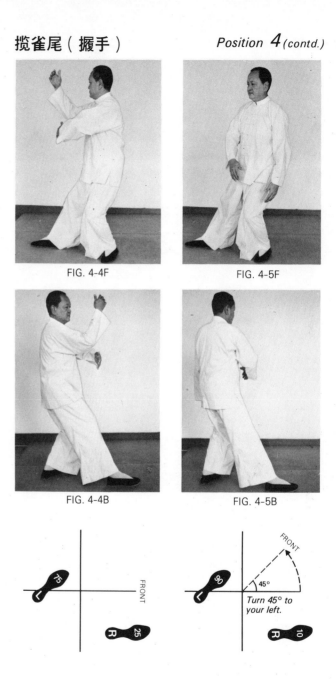

FIG. 4-4F

FIG. 4-5F

FIG. 4-4B

FIG. 4-5B

Turn 45° to your left.

Shift weight to back (L) foot.

揽雀尾（挤手）

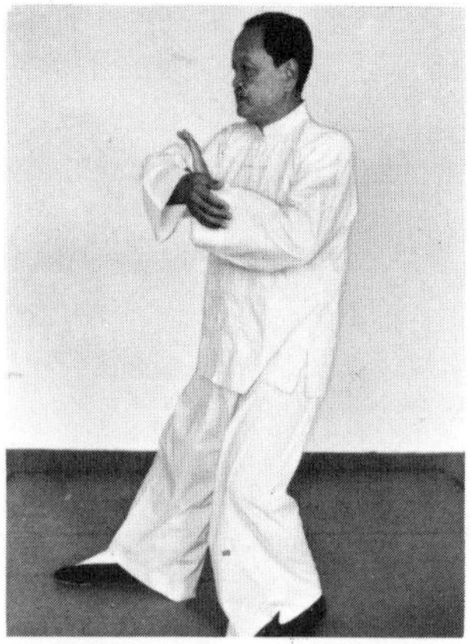

FIG. 4-6F

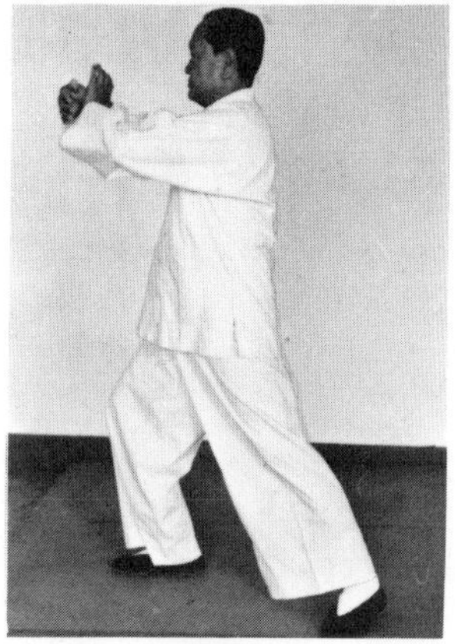

FIG. 4-7F

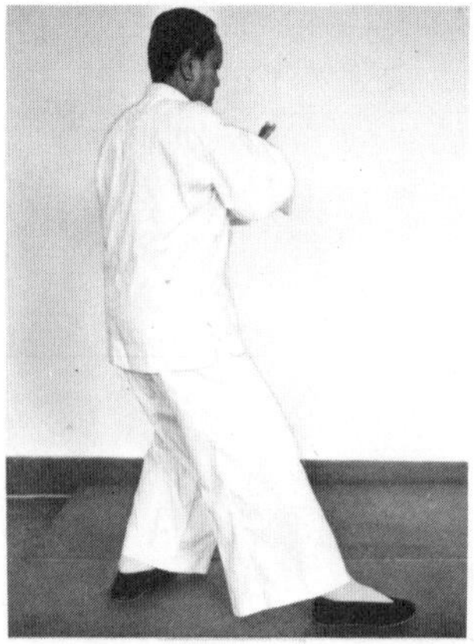

FIG. 4-6B

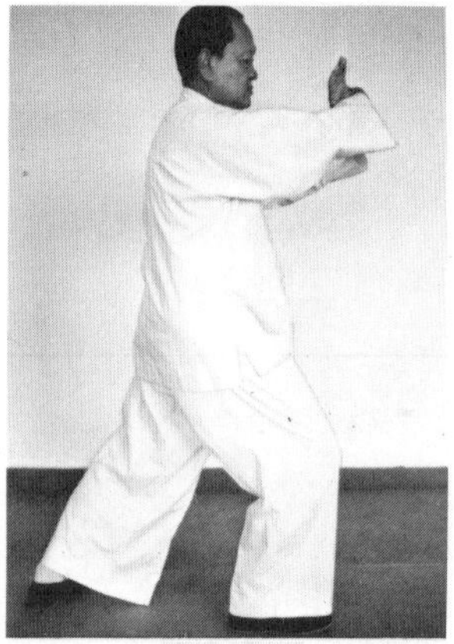

FIG. 4-7B

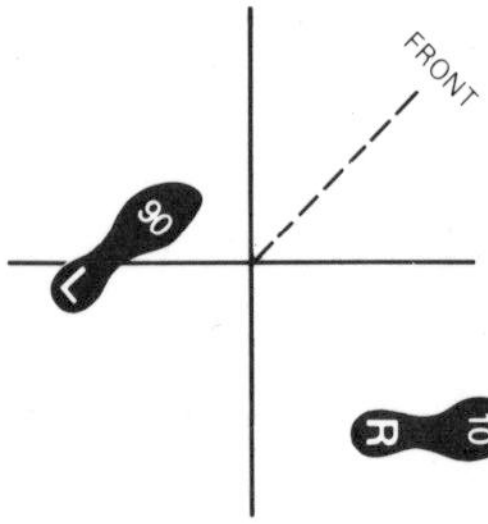

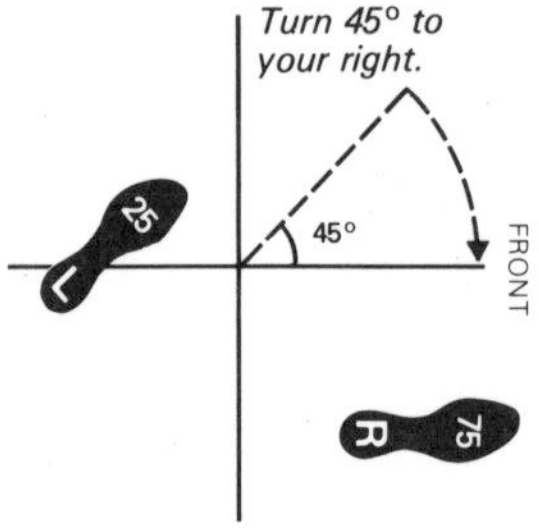

Move forward. Transfer weight to front (R) foot.

Lǎn què wěi (jǐ shǒu)

Grasp sparrow's tail, press

Jǐ shǒu, the third part of this movement, can also be divided in two. First, only movement of hands is involved. Rotate **(R) shoulder** and raise (R) forearm till it is parallel to the floor. Next flex **(L) elbow** to raise (L) forearm and gently press **(L) palm** against the inner part of (R) wrist. During this movement, keep weight on the back **(L) foot** all the time (Fig. 4–6).

Now turn **body** 45° to the right and move forward so your weight is shifted from back (L) foot to front **(R) foot.** Remember that the turn should involve mainly your **waist** with joined hands passive in front of you. At the end of the move about 75 per cent of your weight should be on the **(R) foot** while both (R) knee and joined hands lie in a straight line above the (R) foot. Note that your **palms** should not be held higher than eye level and no force is exerted by the arms. This can be seen in Fig. 4–7 where Chia holds his hands in a very relaxed manner in front of him, with elbows held way below his wrists.

Lǎn què wěi (àn shǒu)

Grasp sparrow's tail, push down

Àn shǒu, the last part of this movement, involves the synchronisation of hand and body movements.

Initially move backward as far as you can, keeping body straight throughout. Pull in **(R) hip** so that both hips are in line with your shoulders. This last effort of pulling in your (R) hip will be difficult to achieve as it will greatly increase the strain on your (L) leg. At the same time rotate both **shoulders** to move both forearms outward to bring them in line with the shoulders. The elbows, shoulders and hips will all be on the same vertical plane if this is achieved. When forearms are in position, rotate **(R) wrist** so (R) palm faces away from you. Both **palms** now face forward. Adduct both shoulders and allow elbows to fall to either side of your body. Hold forearms upright in front with elbows in line with palms. Focus all your weight on the back **(L) foot** and remember that although there is no force on the front leg, the (R) sole should be kept flat on the ground (Fig. 4–8).

Next move forward and, by straightening the back **(L) leg**, transfer at least 75 per cent of your weight onto the front **(R) foot**. Keep both arms relaxed and move them forward as a unit with the body. Stretch your **shoulders** to thrust your elbows forward and upward. Avoid applying tension on your forearms. Focus the thrust on your elbows, keeping them well below the level of hands (Fig. 4–9).

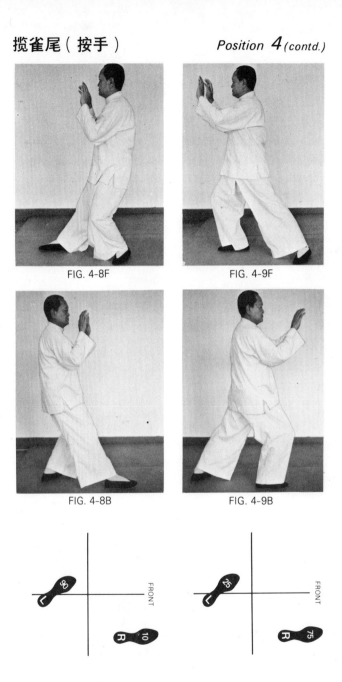

FIG. 4-8F

FIG. 4-9F

FIG. 4-8B

FIG. 4-9B

Move back onto back (L) foot then move forward again onto front (R) foot.

单鞭

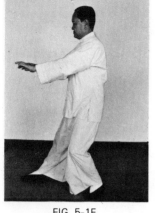

FIG. 5-1F

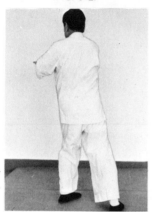

FIG. 5-2F

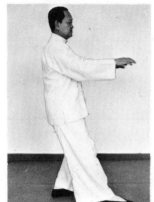

FIG. 5-1B

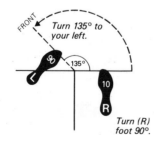

FIG. 5-2B

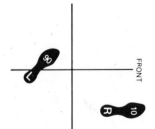

Turn 135° to
your left.

FRONT

135°

10
R

Turn (R)
foot 90°.

Transfer weight to back (L) foot.

Dān biān

Single whip

This is one of the classic postures in tai chi. Over the next few pages we will describe seven link movements that will enable you to move from the last movement, *lǎn què wěi,* to this classic pose.

The first two parts are illustrated on this page. You can see that although there is no overall movement of the body, there is considerable shifting of body weight. First move back and shift weight from front (R) foot to back **(L) foot**. While doing so extend both **elbows** and hold forearms parallel to the floor with **palms** facing downward (Fig. 5–1).

Next turn your **body**, at the waist, 135° to your left while keeping weight focused on **(L) foot**. Do not move (R) foot until you find it difficult to turn further. At this point only, allow **(R) foot** to follow the movement of the body by turning 90° to the left. Your (R) foot should now point straight forward while the (L) foot should point inward. The (L) foot is now at an angle of 45° to the (R) foot (Fig. 5–2).

Dān biān

Single whip

The next three parts of this move also do not involve moving your feet. Move back to bring weight onto back **(R) foot**. Simultaneously flex **(R) elbow** to draw (R) forearm toward you with (R) palm facing downward. Turn **(L) wrist** so the (L) palm now faces the body. Adduct **(L) shoulder** to move **(L) arm** downward and toward you. Keep **(L) elbow** extended so the **(L) palm** faces upward. Both palms now face each other (Fig. 5–3).

Next **turn** 135° to your right. Ensure that you turn at your waist, keeping arms and hands in the same positions in relation to the body with weight concentrated on the **(R) foot** (Fig. 5–4). While you are in this position extend **(R) elbow** to move (R) forearm away from your body until it is in line with (R) upper arm. The entire (R) arm is now perpendicular to your body. When you have completed extending the (R) elbow, flex **(R) wrist** to pull (R) palm downward and hold **(R) thumb** lightly against your second and third fingers. Follow these movements with your eyes (Fig. 5–5).

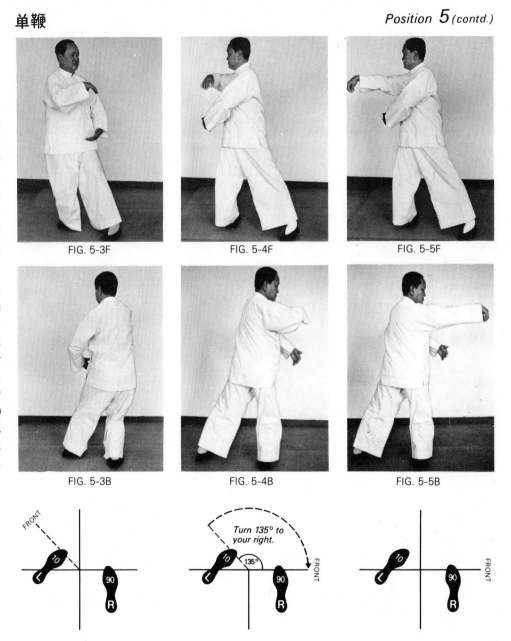

FIG. 5-3F   FIG. 5-4F   FIG. 5-5F

FIG. 5-3B   FIG. 5-4B   FIG. 5-5B

Move back. Transfer weight to (R) foot.

単鞭

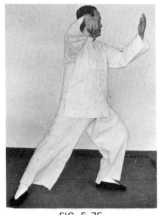

FIG. 5-6F

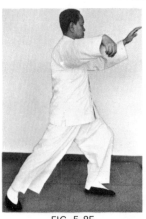

FIG. 5-7F

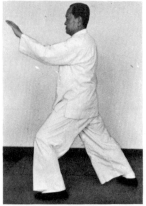

FIG. 5-8F

Dān biān
Single whip

Now rotate **(L) shoulder** so the (L) forearm is raised upright and is in line with the (L) shoulder. Next turn **body** 135° to your left. As you start this turn, lift **(L) heel** off the ground, and with toes resting lightly on the ground pivot on them to turn **(L) foot** and **body** through 135° to your left. The (L) foot should now be perpendicular to the (R) foot. Hold your head up and turn only in conjunction with your body (Fig. 5–6).

Move **(L) foot** forward and outward to the left. Shift weight forward onto **(L) foot** and keep eyes focused on (L) palm (Fig. 5–7). As you move forward turn another 45° to your left so you now face squarely the direction the (L) foot is pointing. Straighten **(R) leg** slightly and turn **(R) foot** 45° to your left. This will bring most of your weight onto the front (L) foot. As you complete the turn rotate **(L) wrist** so that the (L) palm now faces forward. Extend to partially straighten **(L) forearm** and spread **(L) fingers** apart. Your (L) elbow should now lie in front of you and in line with your palm and shoulder. Keep your body as straight as possible. An imaginary line can be drawn through Chia's body from his head to the centre of his pelvis (Fig. 5–8).

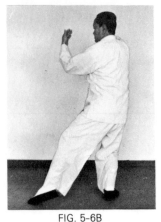

FIG. 5-6B

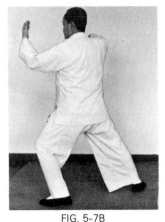

FIG. 5-7B

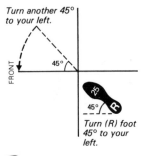

FIG. 5-8B

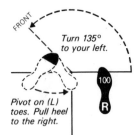

Turn 135° to your left.

Pivot on (L) toes. Pull heel to the right.

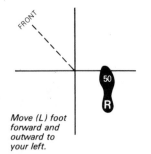

Move (L) foot forward and outward to your left.

Turn another 45° to your left.

45°

45°

Turn (R) foot 45° to your left.

Move forward. Put weight on front (L) foot.

Tí shǒu (shàng shì)

Lift hands, lean forward

Tí shǒu is made up of two separate and distinct movements with the first (*shàng shì*) described below.

From your last move (*dān biān*) which ended with most of your weight on the front (**L**) **foot**, continue loading (L) foot till it carries all your weight. Then **turn** 90° to your right and lift (**R**) **heel** so that only (R) toes lightly touch the ground. Pivot lightly on (R) toes and pull (**R**) **heel** inward until it is in line with toes. Next move both arms concurrently. Extend (**R**) **wrist** and spread out (R) fingers. Now rotate (**R**) **shoulder** to bring point of (R) elbow down and (R) palm facing your left. Keep (R) elbow below the palm. Simultaneously, turn (**L**) **wrist** so (L) palm faces upward (this is termed *pronation*), then flex (**L**) **elbow** to draw (L) arm toward you. Keep it parallel to the ground and stop when it faces the (R) elbow. You should appear to be pulling a rope from some pulley above you (Fig. 6–1).

Taking care not to lift the (R) foot too high off the ground – preferably not more than 7–8 centimetres – 'slide' (**R**) **foot** toward your left till it is in line with and perpendicular to the (L) foot. The (**R**) **heel** should now be the only part of the (R) foot on the ground. All your weight should still be concentrated on the back (**L**) **foot**. Remember to hold yourself erect with your hips pulled well in (Fig. 6–2).

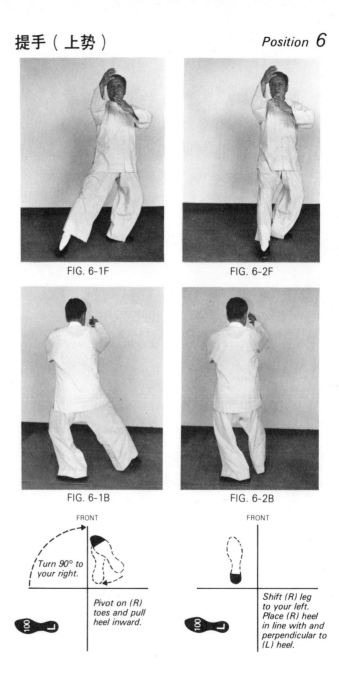

FIG. 6-1F

FIG. 6-2F

FIG. 6-1B

FIG. 6-2B

FRONT

Turn 90° to your right.

Pivot on (R) toes and pull heel inward.

FRONT

Shift (R) leg to your left. Place (R) heel in line with and perpendicular to (L) heel.

Put all your weight on (L) foot.

提手（附靠）

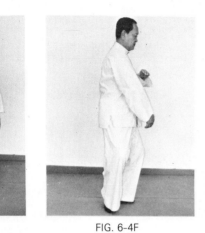

FIG. 6-3F

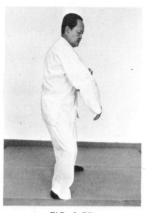

FIG. 6-4F

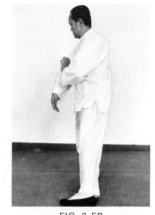

FIG. 6-5F

Tí shǒu (fù kào)

Lift hands, lean forward

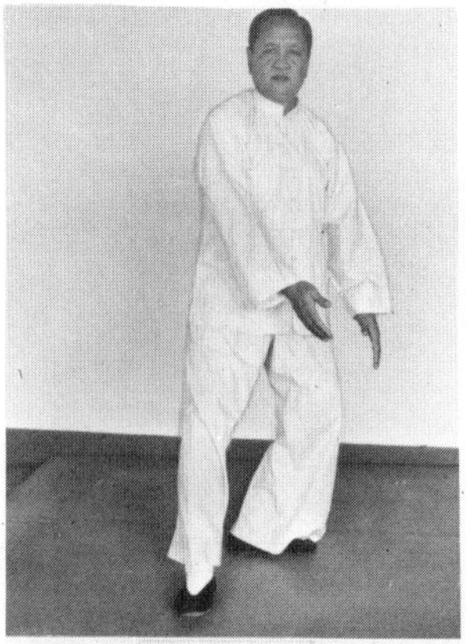

The second part of *tí shǒu (fù kào)* can be described in three separate movements. The first and second involve the lowering and recovery of the arms while the third concerns the moving and shifting of weight onto the front leg.

First adduct both **shoulders** and pull both arms to the left side of your body. Flex **(R) elbow** and pull (R) forearm across your body toward (L) hip. As you carry this out, turn **body** 45° to your left while still keeping your weight on back **(L) foot**. Allow only the heel of (R) foot to be on the ground (Fig. 6-3).

Next flex **(L) elbow** until (L) forearm comes up to the level of the elbow. Remember to hold elbow well below **(L) palm** which should now face and guard (R) elbow. Pull front **(R) foot** back in a straight line with (L) heel. This time permit only **(R) toes** to make contact with the ground. During this movement all your weight should still be on your back **(L) foot** and the (R) arm is still not moved (Fig. 6-4).

Now move **(R) foot** straight out and place it flat on the ground as far forward as is comfortable for you. When you position your feet remember the (R) heel should be placed on the ground before the other parts of your foot. The (R) foot should now be perpendicular to the (L) foot. Having done this, move forward and concentrate at least 75 per cent of your weight on the front **(R) foot** by partially straightening (L) leg. While accomplishing this, remember neither to turn your body nor to move hands in relation to body (Fig. 6-5).

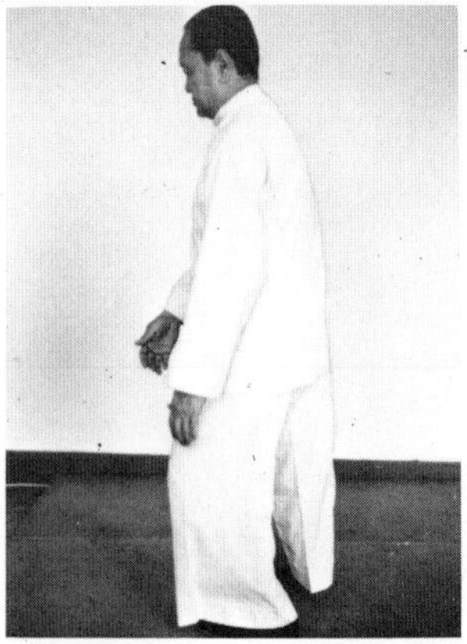

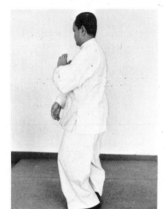

FIG. 6-3B

FIG. 6-4B

FIG. 6-5B

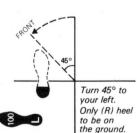

FRONT

45°

100 L

Turn 45° to your left. Only (R) heel to be on the ground.

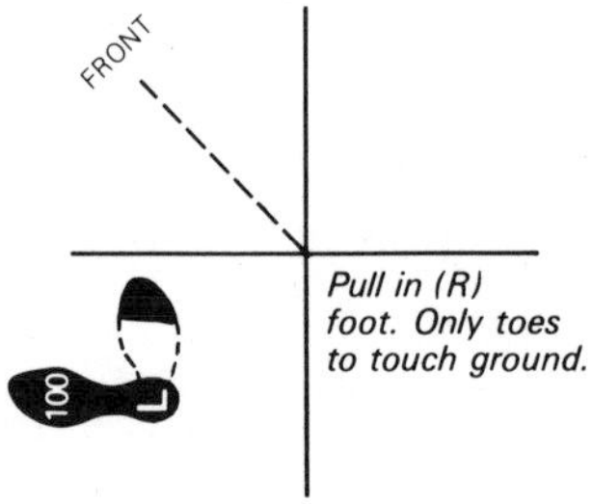

FRONT

100 L

Pull in (R) foot. Only toes to touch ground.

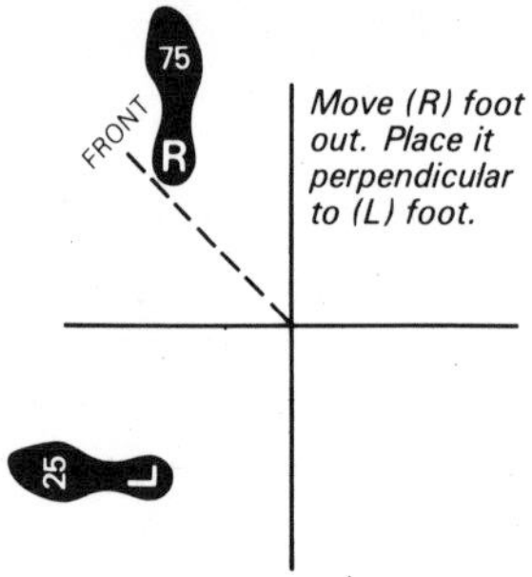

75

R

FRONT

25 L

Move (R) foot out. Place it perpendicular to (L) foot.

Shift weight to (R) foot.

Bái hè liàng chì

White crane spreads wings

This movement can be described in three parts. First, while keeping your weight on the front (R) foot, turn **body** 45° to the right. Do not move either hands or feet at this stage (Fig. 7–1).

Next transfer all your weight onto front **(R) foot** and lift back **(L) leg** slightly off the ground. Bring (L) leg forward and hold it suspended near (R) heel. At the same time abduct **(R) shoulder** and raise (R) upper arm to shoulder level. Then rotate **(R) shoulder** to lift (R) forearm till it is level with (R) shoulder and parallel to the ground. Simultaneously, extend **(L) elbow** and allow (L) forearm to fall by your side with the palm facing downward. Synchronise movements of both arms so the slow upward movement of (R) arm is balanced by the downward movement of (L) forearm (Fig. 7–2).

Complete the move by **turning** 90° to your left and moving **(L) foot** forward in a straight line. Make sure both hips are well pulled in and in line with shoulders. Keep entire weight on back **(R) foot** and permit only toes of (L) foot to touch the ground. In this position, rotate **(R) wrist** so (R) palm now faces outward, away from you. Hold **(L) arm** slightly bent so the (L) palm is by the knee, facing downward. You would, by the end of this move, have struck the posture of a stork unfurling its wings as it prepares to fly away (Fig. 7–3).

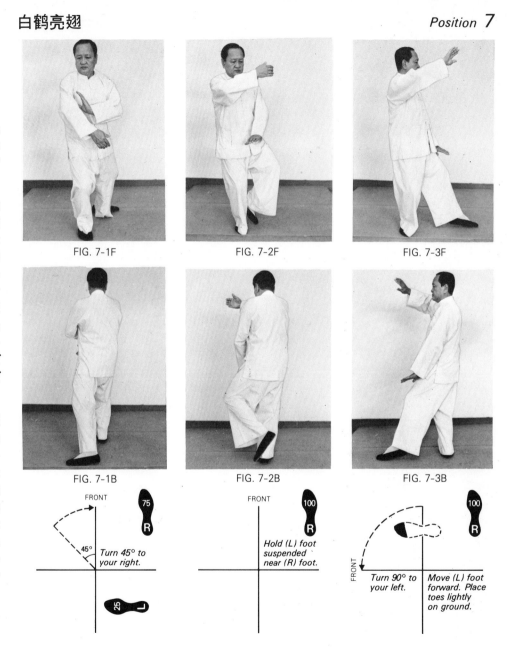

FIG. 7-1F   FIG. 7-2F   FIG. 7-3F

FIG. 7-1B   FIG. 7-2B   FIG. 7-3B

FRONT

75
R

45° *Turn 45° to your right.*

25
L

FRONT

100
R

Hold (L) foot suspended near (R) foot.

100
R

FRONT

Turn 90° to your left. *Move (L) foot forward. Place toes lightly on ground.*

Keep weight concentrated on front (R) foot.

左搂膝拗步

Zuǒ lǒu xī aǒ bù
Brush left knee and pivot step

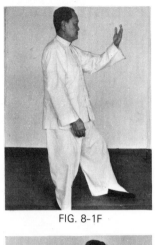

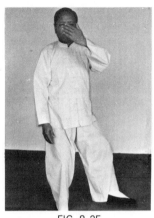

FIG. 8-1F

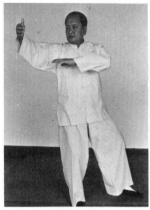

FIG. 8-2F

FIG. 8-3F

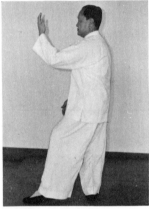

FIG. 8-1B

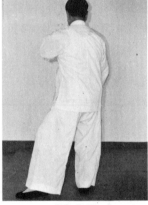

FIG. 8-2B

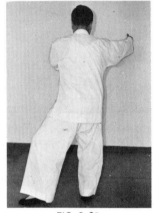

FIG. 8-3B

This movement requires proper coordination of body, hands and feet. Initially only hands are involved. Note that in the three postures shown on this page, all the weight of the body is concentrated on the back **(R) foot** and only the toes of the (L) foot are on the ground.

First adduct and relax **(R) shoulder** to allow (R) arm to fall by your side. At the same time rotate **(L) wrist** to face (L) palm upward, then abduct **(L) shoulder** to raise (L) arm. Keep **(L) elbow** slightly extended so that both the fore and upper (L) arm are raised until the palm is at eye level and is facing you. Keep (L) arm relaxed and flexed at the elbow (Fig. 8–1).

Now turn **body** 45° to your right. Turn **(L) wrist** to your right and rotate (L) shoulder to bring (L) forearm from a vertical to a horizontal position with (L) palm facing downward (Fig. 8–2). Next adduct **(R) shoulder** to raise (R) arm sideways. Keep **(R) elbow** extended so (R) arm is now perpendicular to body (Fig. 8–3).

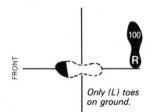

FRONT — 100 R — Only (L) toes on ground.

FRONT — 45° — 100 R — Turn 45° to your right.

FRONT — 100 R — Only (L) toes to touch the ground.

Keep all your weight on back (R) foot.

Zuǒ lǒu xī aǒ bù

Brush left knee and pivot step

Now flex **(R) elbow** to pull (R) forearm inward with (R) palm directly in front of your face (Fig. 8–4).

Next move front **(L) foot** slightly outward and forward. Place (L) heel where (L) toes were (Fig. 8–5). Move forward and begin transferring your weight from back (R) foot to front **(L) foot**. Synchronise this shift of body weight with arm movements. Extend **(L) elbow** and let (L) forearm sweep downward so it lies just beside (L) knee. At the same time adduct **(R) shoulder** to pull (R) elbow downward and forward (Fig. 8–6).

Finally turn **body** 45° to your left, by this time shifting at least 75 per cent of your weight onto front **(L) foot**. The back **(R) foot** should also turn 45° together with your body. While making this turn ensure that (R) foot is kept flat on the ground and is not partially lifted off the ground. At the same time rotate **(R) wrist** so the (R) palm now faces forward. Continue movement of (R) arm by abducting the **(R) shoulder** to push (R) arm in front of you. Concentrate the force on the elbow and not the forearm. Remember to extend **fingers** so they are held in line with (R) wrist and apart from each other. Pull in spine to keep body straight (Fig. 8–7).

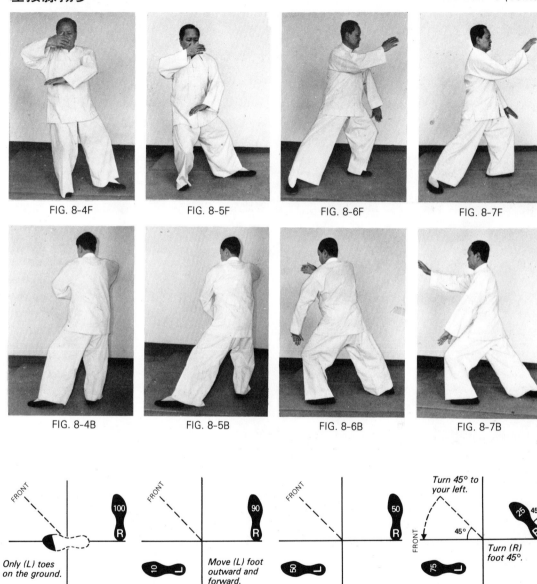

FIG. 8-4F　　FIG. 8-5F　　FIG. 8-6F　　FIG. 8-7F

FIG. 8-4B　　FIG. 8-5B　　FIG. 8-6B　　FIG. 8-7B

Shift weight to front (L) foot.

手挥琵琶

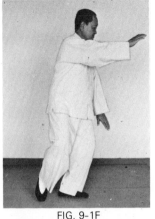

FIG. 9-1F

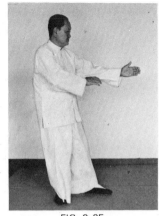

FIG. 9-2F

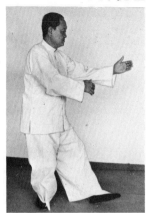

FIG. 9-3F

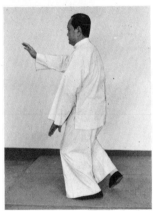

FIG. 9-1B

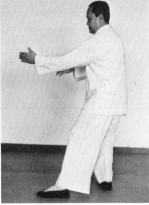

FIG. 9-2B

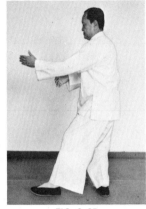

FIG. 9-3B

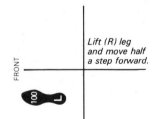

Lift (R) leg and move half a step forward.

FRONT

Leave only (L) toes on ground.

FRONT

Move (L) leg inward till it is in line with (R) heel. Only (L) heel to rest on ground.

FRONT

Shift weight to back (R) foot.

Shǒu huī pí pa

Play the pipa

This position has often been described as 'a man holding a guitar'. First bring entire weight to bear on front **(L) foot** by moving forward and lifting (R) leg slightly off the ground. Move (R) leg half a step forward. Do not attempt to move hands yet (Fig. 9-1).

Next put **(R) foot** down, at right angles to the (L) foot. Move back and shift all your weight onto back **(R) foot.** Lift **(L) foot** slightly, move it forward and allow only the toes to touch the ground. Simultaneously, move both arms. Keep **(L) elbow** extended and abduct **(L) shoulder** till entire (L) arm is parallel to the ground. Extend **(L) fingers** so they point forward. Make sure fingers are held apart from each other. Note the arm is held loosely and slightly bent at the elbow. At the same time, adduct **(R) shoulder** to pull (R) upper arm toward you. Keep **(R) elbow** extended: this will bring (R) hand below (L) elbow. Now rotate **(R) wrist** so (R) palm faces you (Fig. 9-2).

Keeping entire weight on back **(R) foot,** move **(L) foot** to your right and align the heels of both feet so that they point at an angle of 90° to each other. This time place only the **(L) heel** on the ground and ensure that you put no weight on it (Fig. 9-3).

Zuǒ lǒu xī aǒ bù

Brush left knee and pivot step

This is essentially a repetition of the eighth movement (pages 34–35). While keeping your weight on the back **(R) foot,** flex **(L) elbow** to pull (L) forearm upright with (L) palm facing you. Simultaneously, adduct **(R) shoulder** and allow (R) arm to fall by your side (Fig. 10–1).

Turn **body** 45° to your right. Turn **(L) wrist** 90° to your right and then rotate **(L) shoulder** so (L) forearm will be parallel to the ground with **(L) palm** facing downward (Fig. 10–2). Now extend **(R) shoulder** and raise (R) arm sideways till it reaches shoulder level. Keep **eyes** on (R) palm and focus weight on your back **(R) foot.** Note that throughout these three moves the **(L) heel** and not (L) toes rests on the ground (Fig. 10–3).

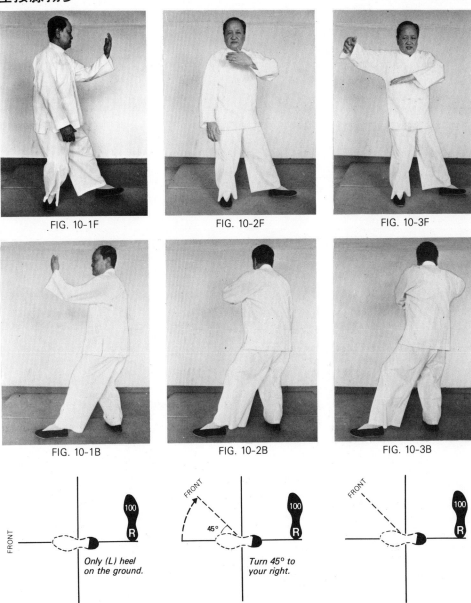

FIG. 10-1F　　　　FIG. 10-2F　　　　FIG. 10-3F

FIG. 10-1B　　　　FIG. 10-2B　　　　FIG. 10-3B

FRONT

Only (L) heel on the ground.

Turn 45° to your right.

FRONT

100 R

Keep entire weight on back (R) foot.

左搂膝拗步

Zuǒ lǒu xī aǒ bù

Brush left knee and pivot step

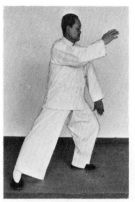

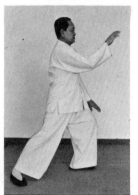

FIG. 10-4F   FIG. 10-5F   FIG. 10-6F   FIG. 10-7F

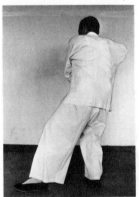

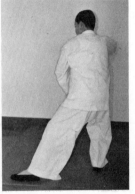

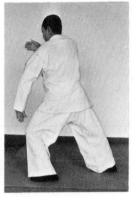

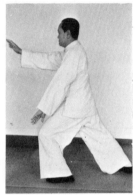

FIG. 10-4B   FIG. 10-5B   FIG. 10-6B   FIG. 10-7B

This is the second part of the movement. A description on how it should be carried out is given on page 35. One thing to note as you move the front (**L**) **foot** is that it should be moved both forward and outward. Be careful not to spread legs too far apart. Then, before you shift your weight forward, make sure your foot is placed flat on the ground.

At the end of the move, when you have shifted your weight onto the front (L) foot, pull in (**L**) **hip** and turn your **waist** so you now face squarely the direction of your front (L) foot. (One quick way to check whether you have done this correctly is to see that hips are in line with your shoulders and (**R**) **palm** is directly in front of the centre of your chest with (**R**) **elbow** relaxed and slightly bent.) Extend (R) arm by stretching shoulder joint. The force that is required for this should be focused on the elbow, not the forearm.

Another common error is the involuntary lifting of the back (R) sole off the ground. This often occurs when you try to assume the correct posture by turning hips completely to your left. One way to overcome this is to ensure that the back (**R**) **knee** is bent slightly with the kneecap pointing toward the toes. Notice that Chia holds his body so straight at the completion of this move that an imaginary line can be drawn from the top of his head through the centre of his pelvis (Fig. 10–7).

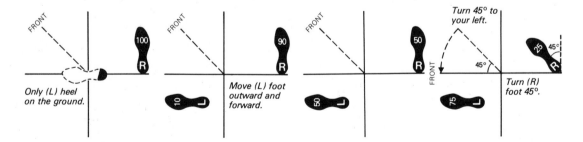

Shift weight to front (L) foot.

Jìn bù, bān, lán chuí

Step forward, deflect downward, parry and punch

This movement can be described in three parts. The first, as its name implies, involves moving straight forward (*jìn bù* – to go forward).

Settle back, bringing nearly all your weight onto the back **(R) foot.** Keep both hands as they were in the last position. As you move back, move entire body as one complete unit, as far as you can. Try to avoid moving either buttocks or upper part of body first. Keep body straight and look forward at the end of the move. This is well illustrated in Fig. 11-1.

Next turn front **(L) foot** 90° to the left, pivoting it on the heel. Do not lift (L) foot off the ground. Clench **(R) hand** and make it into a fist while simultaneously shifting a little of your weight onto your front **(L) foot.** Do not move (L) hand at this point but keep it loose and relaxed near (L) knee (Fig. 11-2).

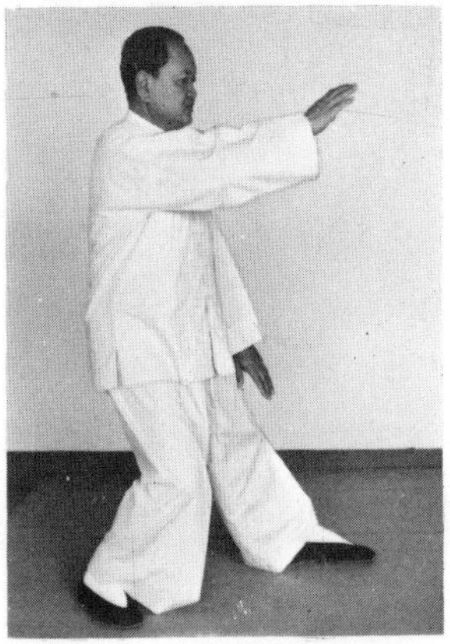

FIG. 11-1F

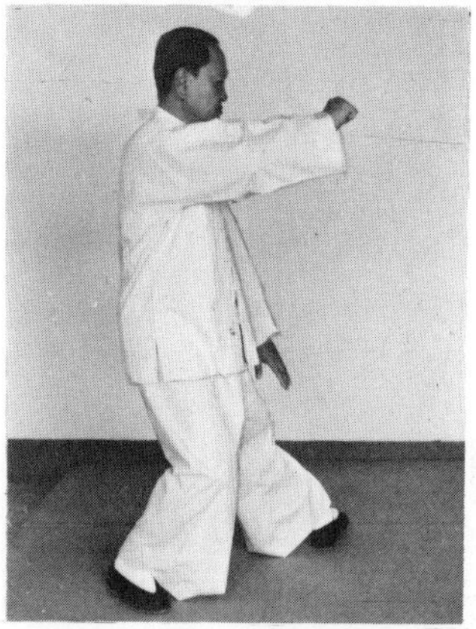

FIG. 11-2F

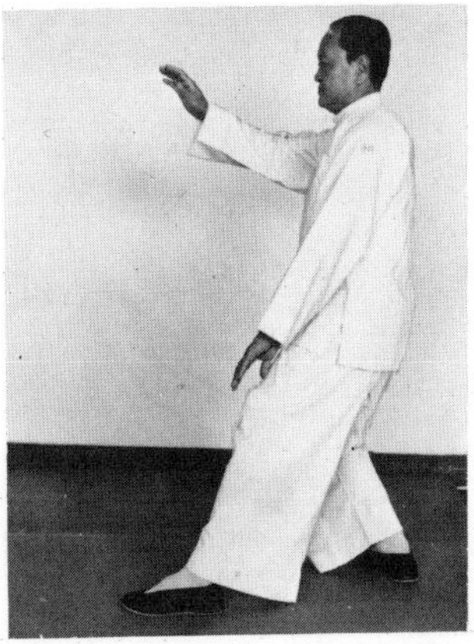

FIG. 11-1B

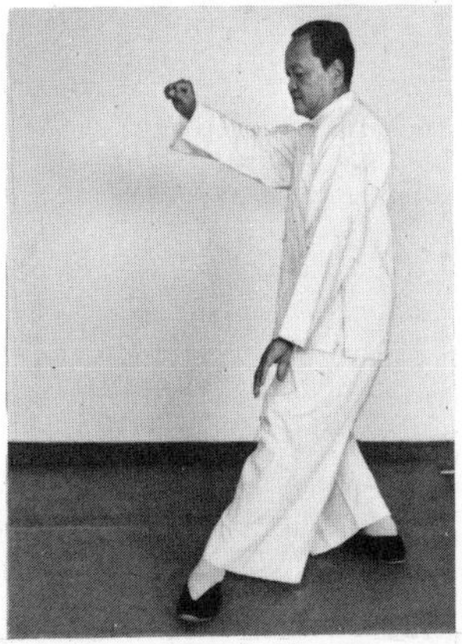

FIG. 11-2B

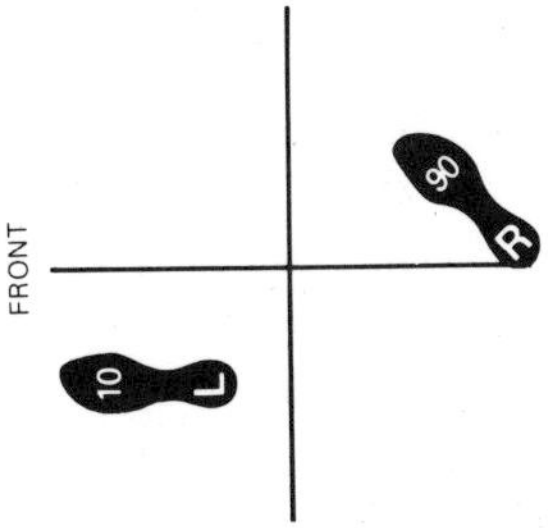

FRONT

90 R

10 L

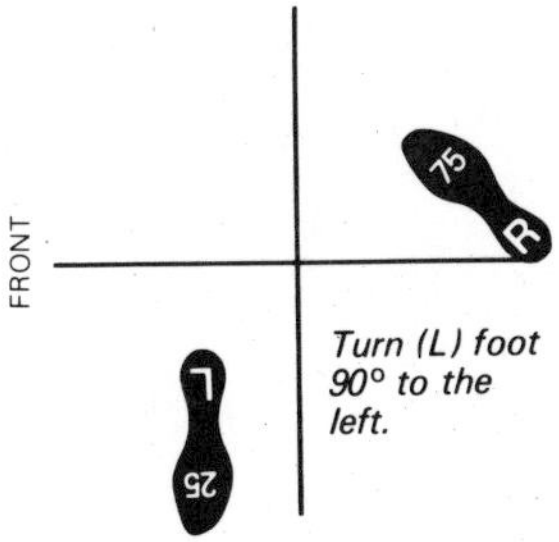

FRONT

75 R

25 L

Turn (L) foot 90° to the left.

Move back. Weight concentrated on back (R) foot.

进步搬拦捶

Jìn bù, bān, lán chuí
Step forward, deflect downward, parry and punch

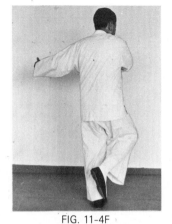

FIG. 11-3F

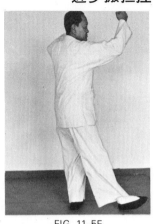

FIG. 11-4F

FIG. 11-5F

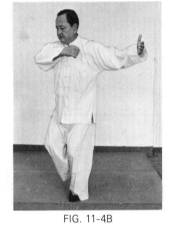

FIG. 11-3B

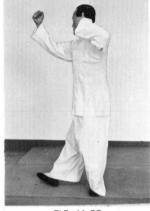

FIG. 11-4B

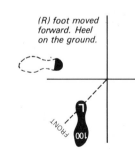

FIG. 11-5B

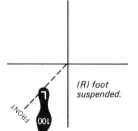

Only (R) toes on the ground.

Turn 45° to your left.

45°

FRONT

100

(R) foot suspended.

FRONT

100

(R) foot moved forward. Heel on the ground.

FRONT

100

The three postures here illustrate the second part (*bān*) of this movement.

First step forward, raising **(R) heel** off the ground and shifting all your weight onto front **(L) foot.** Note that in Fig. 11-3, Chia's back (R) foot carries no weight as only the toes remain in contact with the ground. To avoid raising yourself higher as you straighten (R) foot, bend **(L) knee.** Simultaneously, **turn** 45° to your left and adduct **(R) shoulder** to bring the clenched (R) fist to your side (Fig. 11-3).

Next lift back **(R) foot,** bring it forward and hold it suspended near front (L) heel. At the same time abduct **both shoulders** to raise upper parts of both arms till elbows are in line with shoulders. Keep **(L) elbow** extended so that the abduction of (L) shoulder will raise entire (L) arm sideways. Then flex **(R) elbow** to bring forearm toward you with palm facing the centre of your chest (Fig. 11-4).

Move **(R) foot** straight outward and allow only **(R) heel** to make contact with the ground. Keep weight concentrated on back **(L) foot.** Hold **(R) fist** clenched and extend **(R) elbow** so (R) forearm is now perpendicular to the ground and in line with (R) shoulder. Flex **(L) elbow** at the same time so (L) forearm is pulled toward the body with an open (L) palm lying beside the (L) ear (Fig. 11-5).

Move forward. Transfer weight to front (L) foot.

Jìn bù, bān, lán chuí

Step forward, deflect downward, parry and punch

For this last part of the movement, first pivot **(R) heel** and turn (R) foot 90° to your right. Then straighten back **(L) leg** to shift weight onto front **(R) foot**. Only the toes of the (L) foot should now remain in contact with the ground. As you move forward turn **body** 90° to your right and adduct **(R) shoulder** to allow (R) arm to fall to your side. At the same time rotate then abduct **(L) shoulder** to bring (L) arm forward. Focus your thrust on the (L) elbow and stretch (L) shoulder as far as possible. Keep (L) forearm relaxed. Note that (L) elbow is held well below the palm (Fig. 11–6).

Next move **(L) foot** forward in a straight line. Make sure you do not lift the foot more than a few centimetres off the ground in carrying out this move. Keep your weight on back **(R) foot** (Fig. 11–7).

Now straighten back **(R) leg** to transfer at least 75 per cent of your weight onto front **(L) foot**. As you do this, turn **body** 45° to your left, turn **(R) foot** 45° to the left and pull in **(L) hip** to maintain a straight posture. Move both arms simultaneously with the changes in body position. Flex **(L) elbow** to lower the forearm until the (L) hand is above and beside the (R) elbow. At the same time, with (R) hand still clenched, and keeping (R) elbow extended, abduct **(R) shoulder** to move entire (R) arm forward. Keep the (R) forearm relaxed and parallel to the ground. Do not turn (R) wrist so that the row of knuckles will be perpendicular to the ground. The forward punch with the (R) arm thus involves only (R) shoulder with wrist and elbow held still (Fig. 11–8).

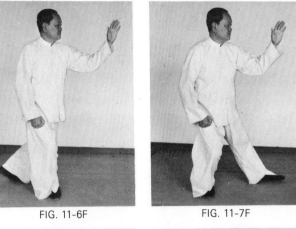

FIG. 11-6F

FIG. 11-7F

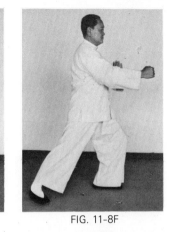

FIG. 11-8F

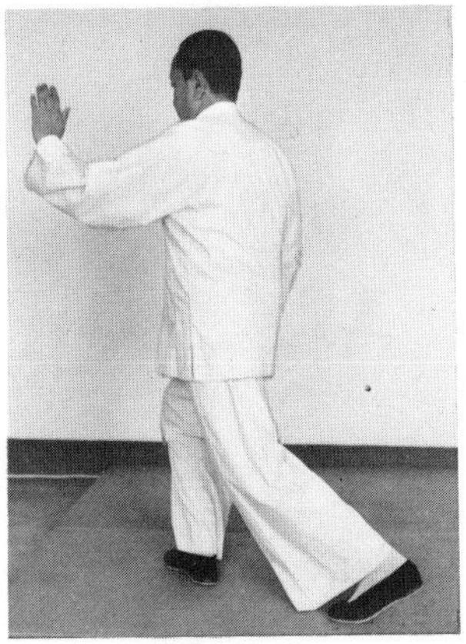

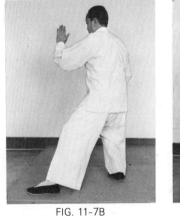

FIG. 11-6B

FIG. 11-7B

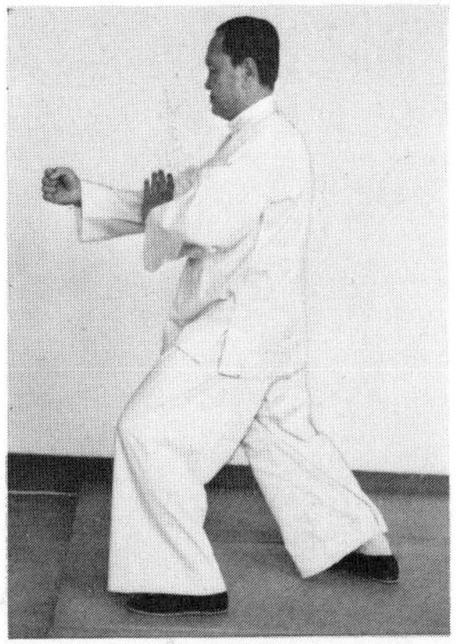

FIG. 11-8B

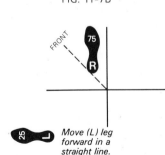

Turn (R) foot 90°.
Turn 90° to your right.
(L) toes on the ground.

Turn (R) foot 90°.
Move (L) leg forward in a straight line.

Turn (R) foot through 45°.
Turn 45° to your left.

Step forward. Transfer weight to (R) foot. Then move forward to bring weight to front (L) foot.

如封似闭

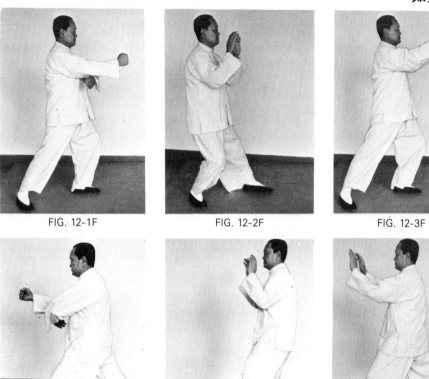

FIG. 12-1F   FIG. 12-2F   FIG. 12-3F

FIG. 12-1B   FIG. 12-2B   FIG. 12-3B

Rú fēng sì bì

Withdraw and push

This move consists essentially of a quick withdrawal followed by an aggressive push forward. First extend (R) elbow a little more and let **(L) palm** fall below (R) elbow. Leave most of your weight on front **(L) foot** at this point (Fig. 12–1).

Now retreat by shifting weight onto back **(R) foot.** Coordinate this with the arm movements. Rotate **(L) shoulder** and bring (L) forearm forward and outward from under (R) arm. If you had moved only (L) shoulder, the (L) palm should face you at this stage. Next rotate **(L) wrist** so the palm faces outward. Adduct **(L) shoulder** to allow (L) arm, bent at elbow, to sink to the side of the body.

Simultaneously, unclench **(R) fist** and turn **(R) wrist** so the open (R) palm faces outward. Coordinate this movement so both palms face outward at the same time. Next adduct **(R) shoulder** to pull (R) elbow to your side. Both forearms should now be upright with palms facing outward (Fig. 12–2).

Finally straighten back **(R) leg** to shift weight onto front **(L) foot.** As you carry this out abduct **both shoulders** to push both arms out. The thrust of this move should be concentrated in your elbows. Both forearms should be relaxed. Remember to keep your **body** straight (Fig. 12–3).

Move back then forward to shift weight to front (L) foot.

Shí zì shǒu

Cross hands

This move follows immediately after the last. Many tend to pause at this point: you must try to avoid this error.

Shift your weight onto the back **(R) foot.** As you move backward, extend both arms to stretch your shoulders. One thing to look out for in executing this move is to avoid moving your **body** backward at a slant. (In combat, this is not good practice as your opponent can take advantage of your improper stance to upset your balance.) Another point to note is to ensure that the **(R) knee** is bent when you move back as this will allow you to maintain a level height and to focus your weight onto the back (R) foot (Fig. 13–1).

Once you have moved back fully, turn **body** 90° to your right by pivoting on **(L) heel.** The **(L) foot** should also follow by turning 90°. This is only possible if all your weight is on the **(R) foot.** As you turn abduct both **shoulders** till the arms are in line with your body and both **palms** face outward, away from the body (Fig. 13–2).

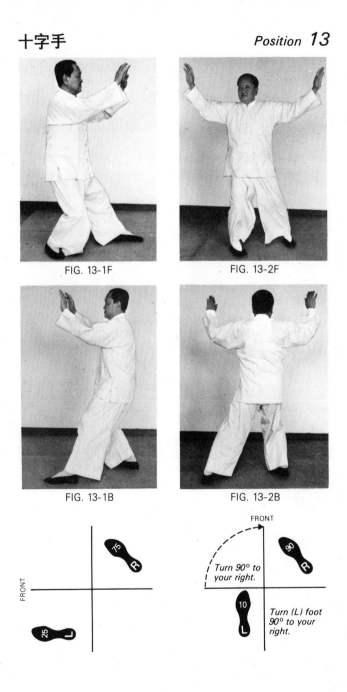

FIG. 13-1F

FIG. 13-2F

FIG. 13-1B

FIG. 13-2B

FRONT

75 R

FRONT

25 L

FRONT

Turn 90° to your right.

90 R

10 L

Turn (L) foot 90° to your right.

Move back. Transfer weight to front (R) foot.

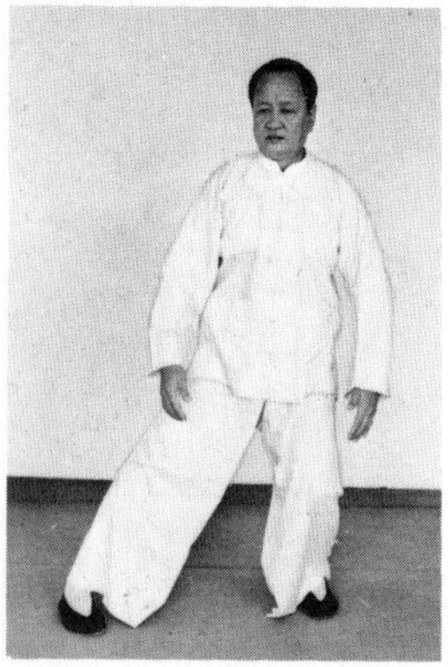

十字手

FIG. 13-3F 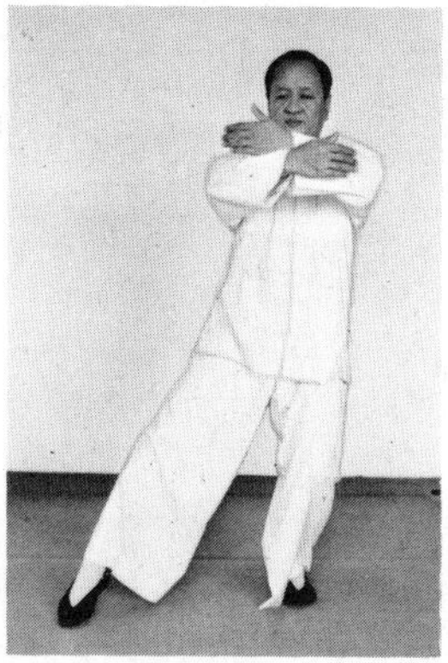   FIG. 13-4F 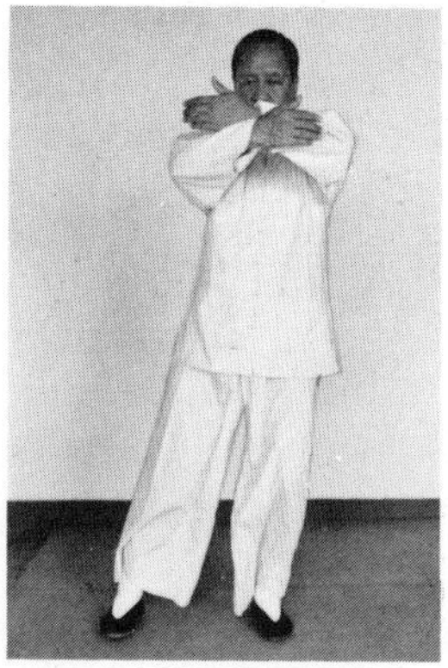   FIG. 13-5F 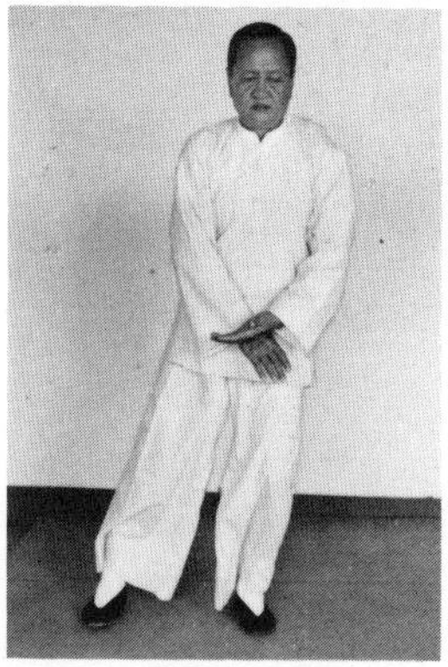   FIG. 13-6F

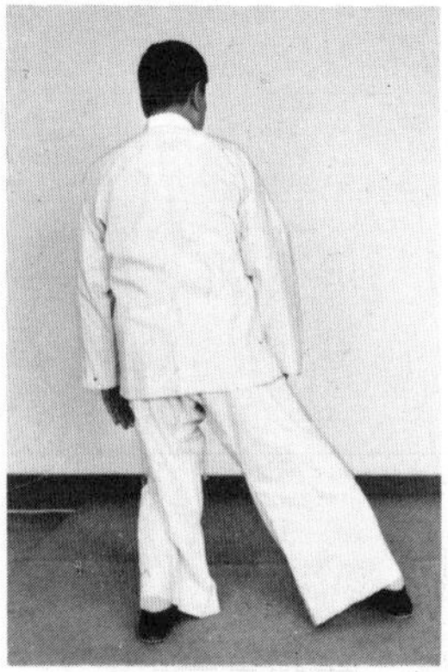

FIG. 13-3B 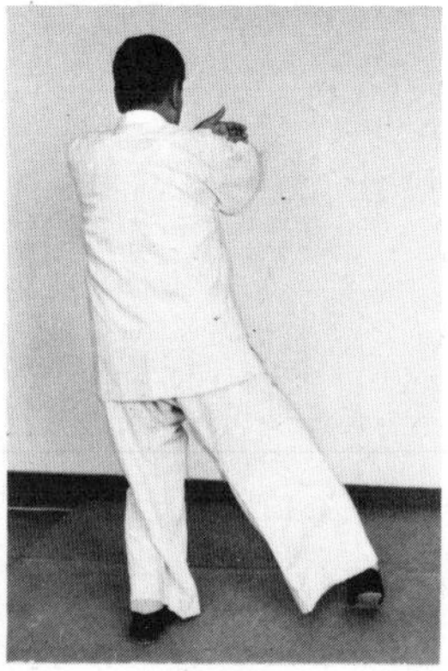   FIG. 13-4B 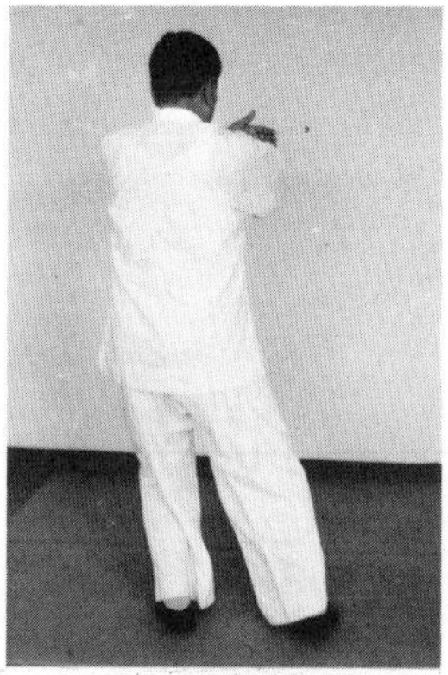   FIG. 13-5B 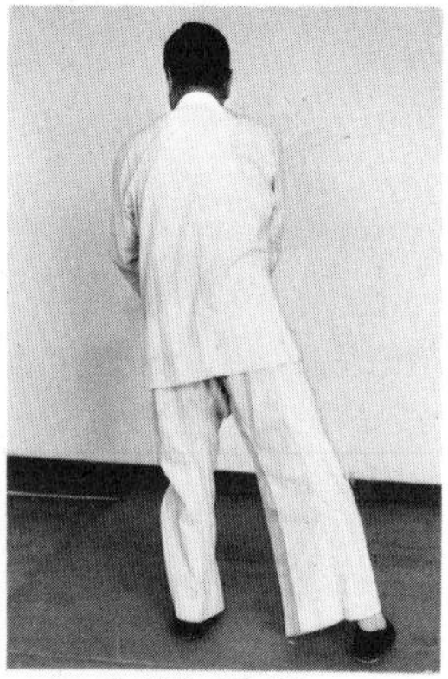   FIG. 13-6B

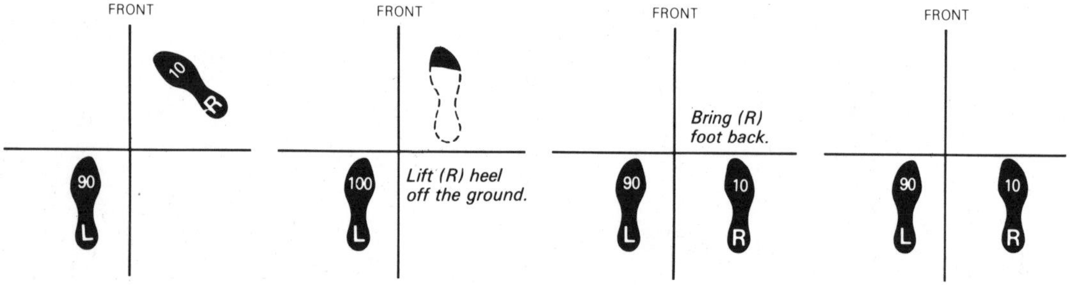

FRONT   FRONT   FRONT   FRONT

Lift (R) heel off the ground.

Bring (R) foot back.

Shift weight to (L) foot.

Shí zì shǒu

Cross hands

Continue the move by shifting weight back to **(L) foot.** At the same time adduct both **shoulders** and then extend both **elbows** simultaneously to permit both arms to fall to your sides. Both **palms** should face inward, toward you (Fig. 13-3).

Next lift **(R) heel** off the ground and pull it to your left till it is in line with toes. Abduct both **shoulders** to lift arms forward. When arms are parallel to the ground rotate **shoulders** so forearms cross in front of you with (R) forearm on the outside of the left. Note that intersection of the forearms is made away from the body (Fig. 13-4).

While keeping both arms in position, pull **(R) foot** back and place it flat on the ground at the same level as (L) foot. Your weight should still be mostly on the **(L) foot** (Fig. 13-5).

Finally adduct **shoulders** and partially extend **elbows** so both arms hang loosely crossed in front of your pelvis. Note that your weight should still be mostly on the **(L) foot** (Fig. 13-6).

This completes Chapter One of the exercise. At this stage, you are advised to review the sequence and moves contained in this chapter until you are reasonably familiar with them, before proceeding to subsequent chapters.

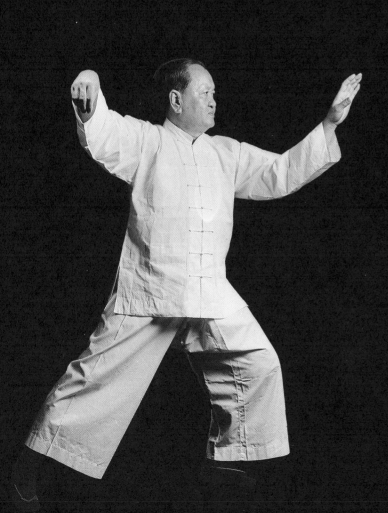

Chapter Two

This marks the beginning of Chapter Two which is relatively short, being made up of seven different moves. However, as these involve several repetitive movements, you will take approximately the same time to complete them as you did the first part.

抱虎归山

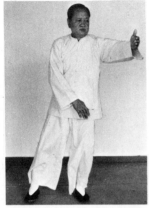

FIG. 14-1F

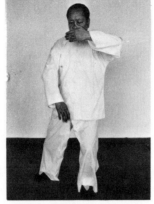

FIG. 14-2F

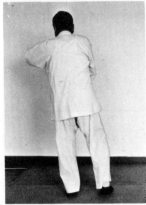

FIG. 14-1B

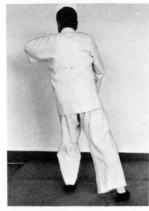

FIG. 14-2B

Bào hǔ guī shān
Embrace tiger and return to mountain

First, while keeping weight mostly on **(L) foot,** abduct **(L) shoulder** to raise (L) arm sideways. Keep **(L) elbow** extended so entire (L) arm is raised till it is at shoulder level and parallel to the floor. Focus **eyes** on (L) palm which should face you at this point. Keep **(R) arm** in the same position, lying passively across your body (Fig. 14–1).

Now move **(R) foot** straight back, keeping toes pointing forward. Both feet should still face the same direction. Concentrate weight on front **(L) foot.** Flex **(L) elbow** and draw (L) forearm toward you with palm facing the centre of your body. Focus eyes on (L) palm (Fig. 14–2).

FRONT

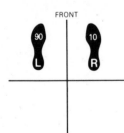

FRONT

Move (R) foot back. Both feet still face the same direction.

Keep weight on (L) foot.

Bào hǔ guī shān

Embrace tiger and return to mountain

Pivot on **(R) heel** and turn (R) foot 135° to your right. Keep weight on the front **(L) foot** otherwise you will lose your balance when you carry out this move. Follow the movement of (R) foot by turning **body** 45° to the right. Do not move the arms. Note that Chia holds his **(R) arm** bent at the elbow and away from his body (Fig. 14–3).

Now gradually shift weight from (L) to **(R) foot** till it eventually carries at least 75 per cent of your weight. Initially turn **body** another 45° to your right and at the same time extend **(R) elbow** to sweep (R) hand across the body till it lies near (R) knee. Do not move **(L) arm** and keep it relaxed, flaccid and bent at the elbow (Fig. 14–4).

Complete the move by turning **body** another 45° to your right. You would now have turned your body 135° to the right to face squarely the direction the (R) foot is pointing. Turn **(L) foot** 45° to the right. It should now lie perpendicular to the (R) foot with both heels in line with each other. Now rotate **(L) shoulder** to bring (L) elbow down, then abduct **(L) shoulder** to move (L) arm forward. Keep **(L) elbow** partially extended. Notice that Chia does not exert any strength in his **(L) forearm**. All force should be directed at the elbow. At this point let **(R) arm** lie passively by (R) knee and keep at least 75 per cent of your weight on front **(R) leg.** Note that **(R) knee** points in the same direction as (R) toes and **eyes** should be focused on (L) palm (Fig. 14–5).

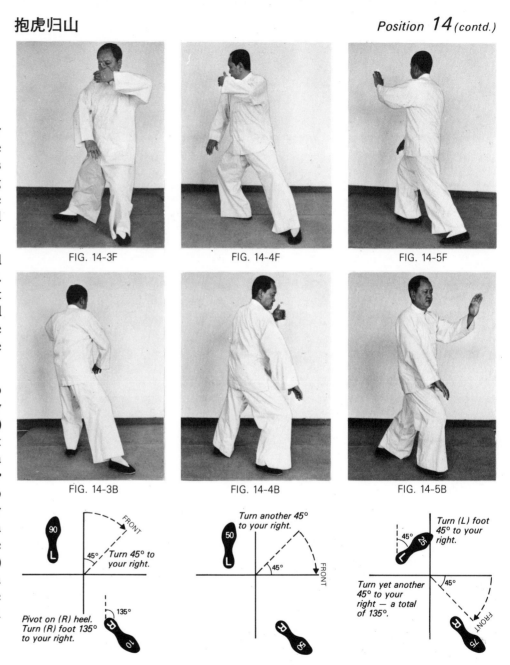

FIG. 14-3F   FIG. 14-4F   FIG. 14-5F

FIG. 14-3B   FIG. 14-4B   FIG. 14-5B

Pivot on (R) heel. Turn (R) foot 135° to your right.

Turn another 45° to your right.

Turn (L) foot 45° to your right.

Turn yet another 45° to your right — a total of 135°.

Gradually shift weight to (R) foot.

抱虎归山

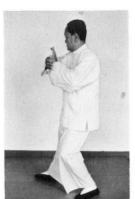

FIG. 14-6F

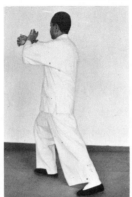

FIG. 14-7F

FIG. 14-8F

FIG. 14-9F

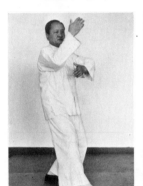

FIG. 14-6B

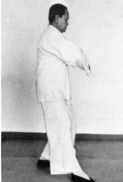

FIG. 14-7B

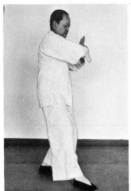

FIG. 14-8B

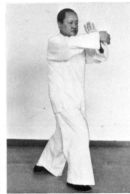

FIG. 14-9B

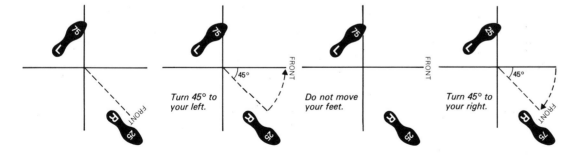

Initially roll back and put weight on back (L) foot.
Then move forward, transferring weight to front (R) foot.

Bào hǔ guī shān
Embrace tiger and return to mountain

The latter part of this move is similar to that described for Position 4 – *lǎn què wěi* (pages 24–27).

The first two parts – *lí shǒu* and *jǐ shǒu* – are illustrated here. Rather than repeat detailed descriptions of these moves, some of their more important aspects will be highlighted here. The essence of these moves lies in the proper synchronisation of turns with the shifting of weight from one foot to the other.

First adduct **(R) shoulder** to raise (R) upper arm then flex **(R) elbow** so (R) forearm is pulled to a vertical position with **(R) palm** facing you. Then turn **(L) wrist** so (L) palm faces you, and flex **(L) elbow.** Bring (L) forearm toward you till **(L) palm** is below **(R) elbow.** As you execute these hand movements shift weight onto back **(L) foot** (Fig. 14-6). When you have moved as far back as you can, turn **body** 45° to your left. At the same time allow (L) arm to fall to your side and rotate **(R) shoulder** so (R) forearm will now lie parallel to the ground (Fig. 14-7).

Abduct **(L) shoulder,** flex **(L) elbow** and then gently press **(L) palm** against inner side of (R) wrist (Fig. 14-8). Finally straighten back **(L) leg,** move forward, **turn** 45° to your right and transfer weight onto front **(R) foot** (Fig. 14-9).

Bào hǔ guī shān

Embrace tiger and return to mountain

The last part of this move is similar to *àn shǒu,* described on page 27. First move back onto **(L) foot,** simultaneously rotating both **shoulders** bringing elbows down and separating hands. Turn **(R) wrist** so both palms now face outward, then adduct **shoulders** to pull arms toward you. Remember that elbows should sink downward but not backward (Fig. 14-10).

Finally straighten back **(L) leg,** move forward and shift at least 75 per cent of your weight onto the front **(R) foot.** The force of this forward thrust should come from the back **(L) foot.** As you move forward keep both **elbows** slightly flexed, and never, ever extend them completely. Stretch **shoulders** to thrust your elbows upward and forward and do not exert any force in your forearms. (Fig. 14-11).

Note that throughout the latter part of this move the emphasis of the moves has been on the turning of your body and the shifting of weight from one leg to the other.

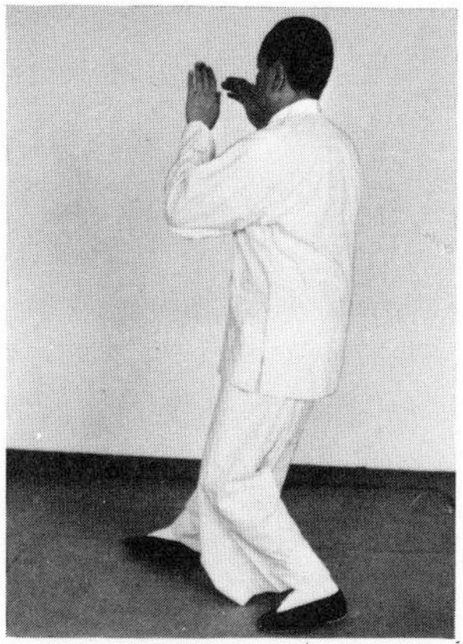

FIG. 14-10F

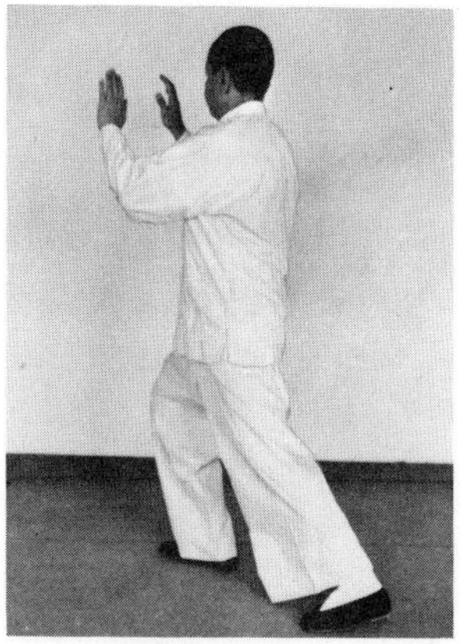

FIG. 14-11F

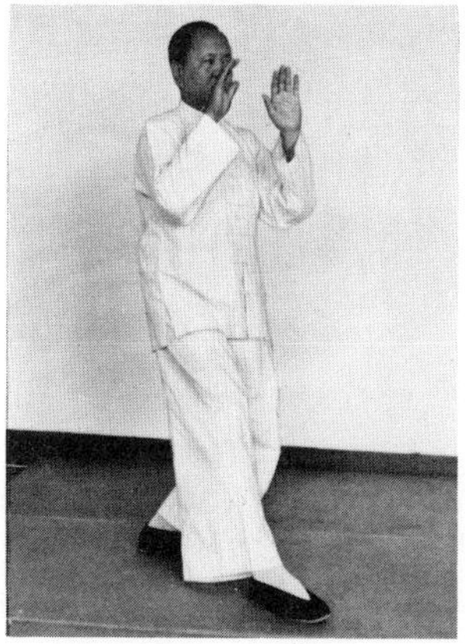

FIG. 14-10B

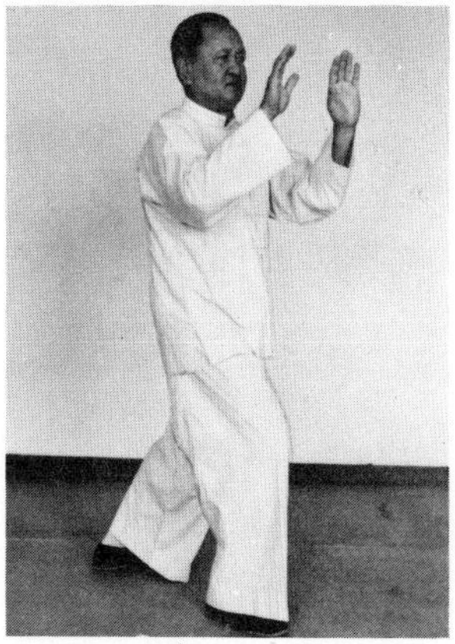

FIG. 14-11B

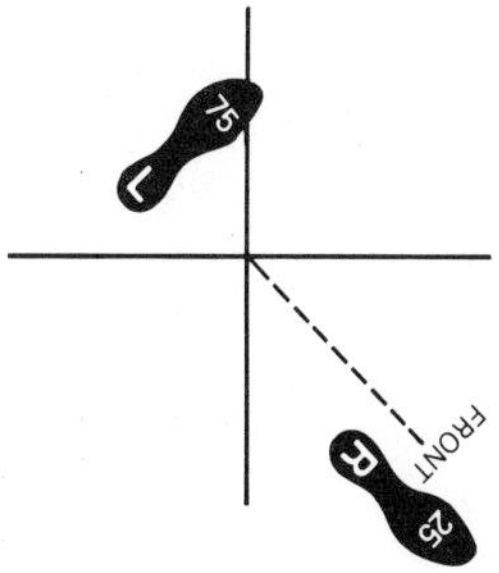

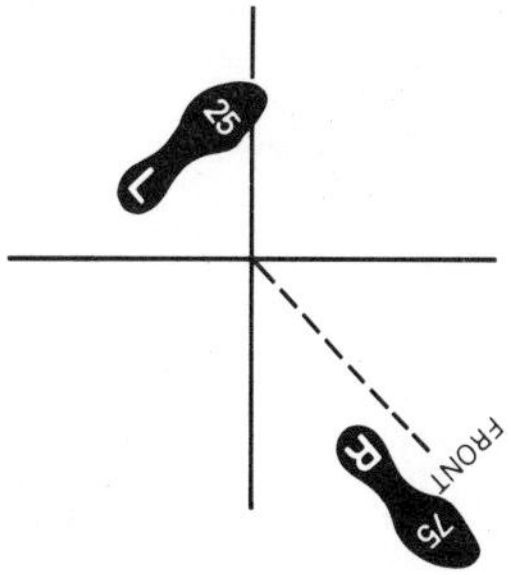

Move back onto (L) foot and then forward, shifting weight to front (R) foot.

斜单鞭

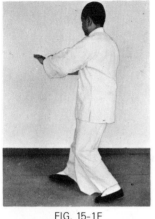

FIG. 15-1F

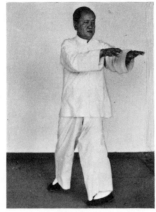

FIG. 15-2F

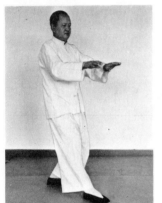

FIG. 15-1B

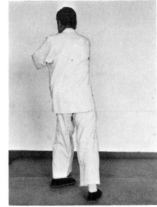

FIG. 15-2B

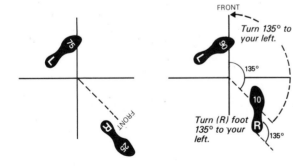

Transfer weight to (L) foot.

Xié dān biān
Diagonal single whip

This is basically similar to Position 5 (*dān biān*) on pages 28–30, except that it is carried out at a different angle. The two pictures here illustrate some of the link movements which bring you from Position 14 *(bào hǔ guī shān)* to this move.

First move back and allow at least 75 per cent of your weight to rest on back **(L) foot.** Extend both **elbows** to drop both forearms simultaneously, until forearms and hands lie parallel to the floor with **palms** facing downward (Fig. 15–1).

As you are settling on the back (L) foot with body held as straight as possible, turn **body** 135° to your left. In order to do this you should first focus all your weight on **(L) foot** and permit **(R) foot** to turn with the body, using the heel as a pivot. The (R) foot should not turn simultaneously with the body but should follow **after** you have initiated the turn. Allow **(R) foot** to turn only when you have difficulty in turning your waist further. The (R) foot should have turned 90° only when you have turned the body 135° in the same direction. Put only minimal weight, about 10 per cent, on (R) foot for wrong weight distribution will impede your turn and will tend to make you fall. Keep both hands passive and permit them to follow the turning of your body (Fig. 15–2).

Xié dān biān

Diagonal single whip

斜单鞭

At the end of the turn, settle back and shift all your weight onto the **(R) foot.** Adduct **(L) shoulder** and keep (L) elbow slightly bent. This will bring (L) arm to your side with **(L) palm** facing upward. Flex **(R) elbow** so **(R)** forearm is pulled toward you with **(R) palm** facing downward. Both palms should now face each other and it would appear that you could hold a ball between them (Fig. 15–3).

Now, while keeping weight on back **(R) foot,** turn **body** 90° to your right. As you accomplish this, do not move feet and try to maintain the same height (Fig. 15–4).

Next, while holding your body in exactly the same position, extend **(R) elbow** and flex **(R) wrist,** pressing thumb lightly against third finger. Remember that the (R) arm should never be tense (Fig. 15–5).

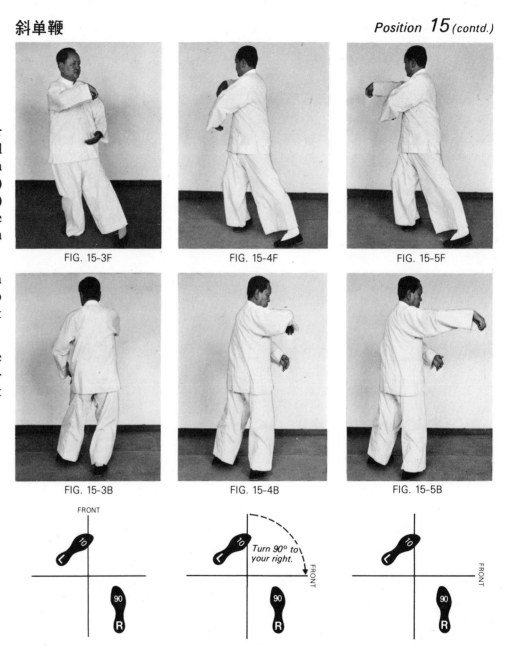

FIG. 15-3F   FIG. 15-4F   FIG. 15-5F

FIG. 15-3B   FIG. 15-4B   FIG. 15-5B

FRONT

Turn 90° to your right.

Move back. Transfer weight to (R) foot.

斜单鞭

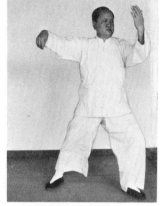

FIG. 15-6F

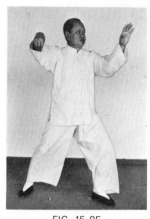

FIG. 15-7F

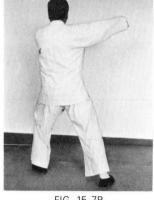

FIG. 15-8F

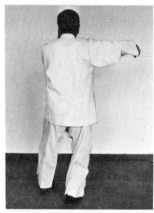

FIG. 15-6B

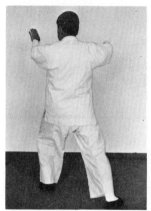

FIG. 15-7B

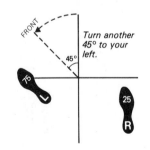

FIG. 15-8B

Xié dān biān

Diagonal single whip

Now, to conclude this move. First, while keeping **(L) elbow** flexed, rotate **(L) shoulder** to lift (L) forearm till **(L) palm** faces you at eye level. Now turn *body* 90° to your left, simultaneously lifting **(L) heel** off the ground in order to pivot easily on (L) toes. Do not move outstretched (R) arm (Fig. 15–6).

The remaining two steps are identical to those described previously for Position 5 (page 30). Instead of repeating ourselves, let us try to refine the final move (Figs. 15–7 and 15–8).

Keep your body as straight as possible. Pull up your coccyx and pull in your stomach to help you attain this position. Your (L) palm, elbow and shoulder should all be in the same straight line with the elbow **below** the level of the palm. Rotate (L) shoulder to turn the point of the elbow till it faces vertically downward. Notice how expansively Chia spreads his arms when he executes this move.

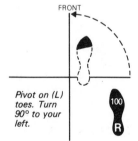

Pivot on (L) toes. Turn 90° to your left.

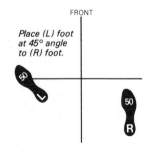

Place (L) foot at 45° angle to (R) foot.

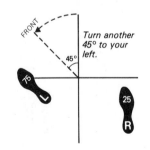

Turn another 45° to your left.

Transfer weight to (L) foot.

Zhǒu dǐ kàn chuí

Punch under elbow

This is a relatively difficult move to execute and is illustrated over nine photographs. The first three are shown here.

The first part involves shifting your weight onto the back **(R) foot.** As you do this lift (L) toes so only **(L) heel** is on the ground (Fig. 16–1).

Next turn **body** 45° to your left, and at the same time abduct **(L) shoulder** and move it sideways to your left, until both arms are in line with each other. Your **(L) palm** should face downward. Simultaneously, rotate **(R) wrist** so **(R) palm** faces forward, in the same direction as your body. Note that both palms face different directions. When you have completed your turn, move **(L) foot** to your left and place (L) heel in line with and perpendicular to (R) heel. All your weight should be concentrated on the **(R) foot** (Fig. 16–2).

Now move forward by straightening back (R) leg until front **(L) foot** takes on at least 75 per cent of your weight. Make sure **(L) knee** does not extend beyond (L) toes and remember to keep **(R) leg** slightly bent with (R) knee pointing toward (R) toes. Notice that both of Chia's palms are still pointing at different directions at this stage (Fig. 16–3).

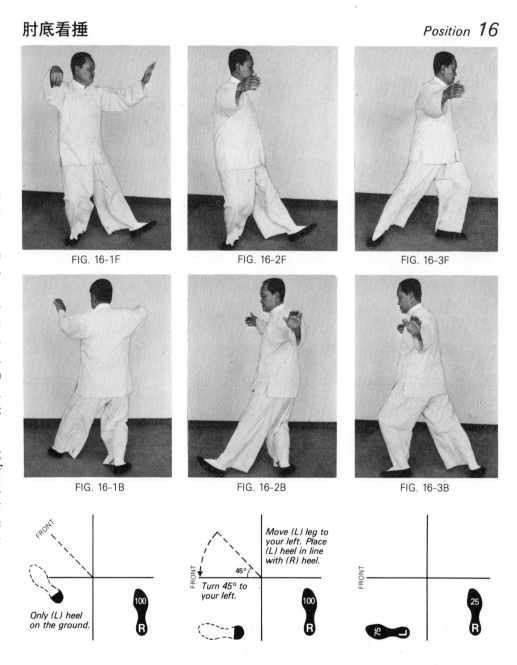

FIG. 16-1F   FIG. 16-2F   FIG. 16-3F

FIG. 16-1B   FIG. 16-2B   FIG. 16-3B

FRONT

Only (L) heel on the ground.

FRONT Turn 45° to your left. 45° Move (L) leg to your left. Place (L) heel in line with (R) heel.

100 R

FRONT 100 R

FRONT 75 L 25 R

Settle back. Then move forward and transfer weight onto front (L) foot.

肘底看捶

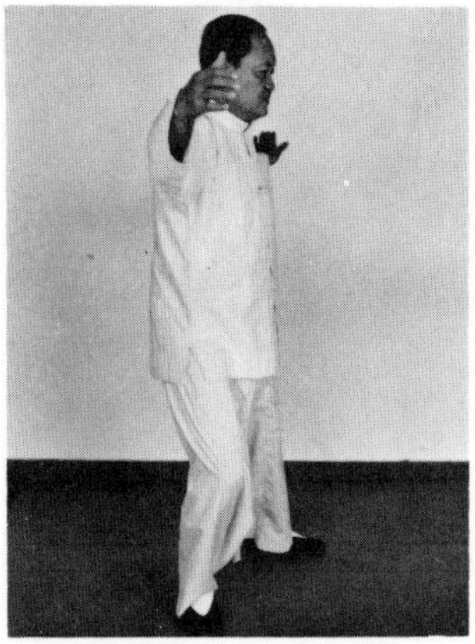

FIG. 16-4F

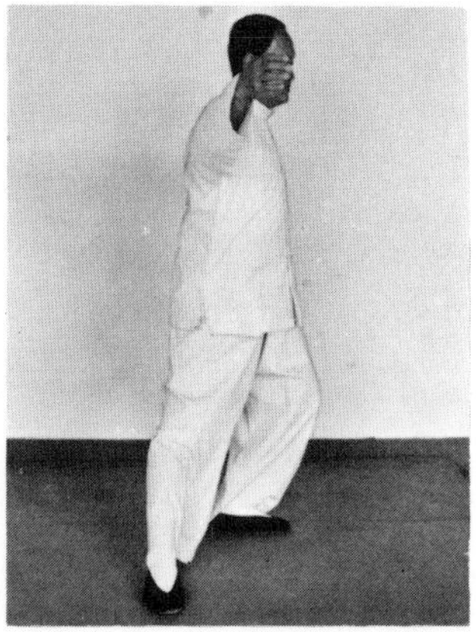

FIG. 16-5F

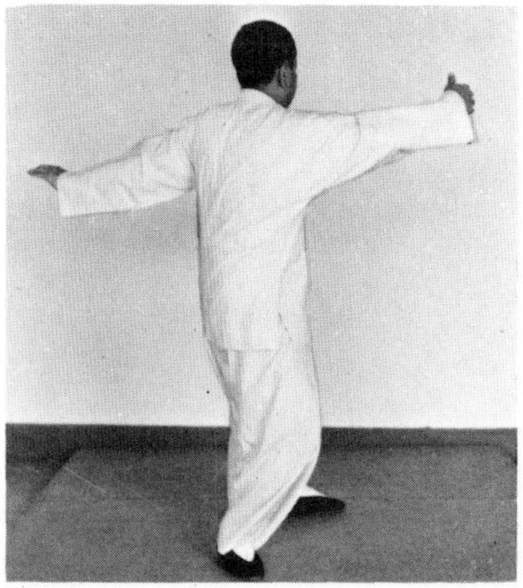

FIG. 16-6F

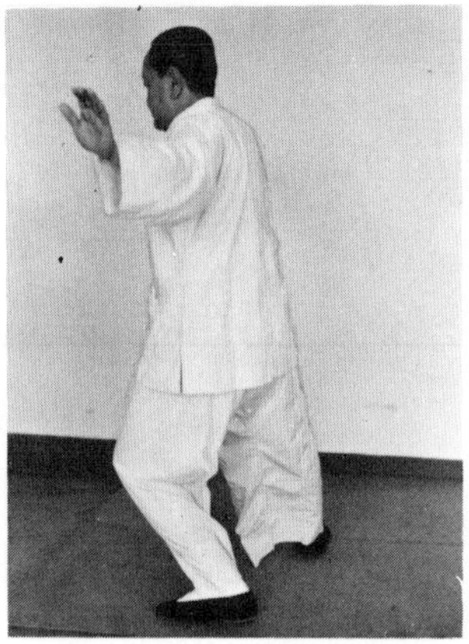

FIG. 16-4B

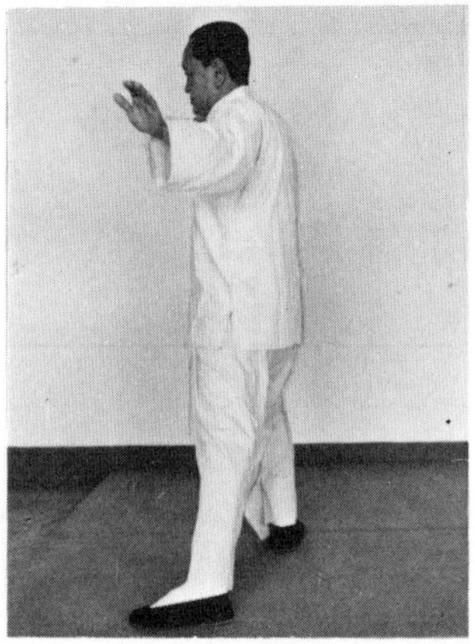

FIG. 16-5B

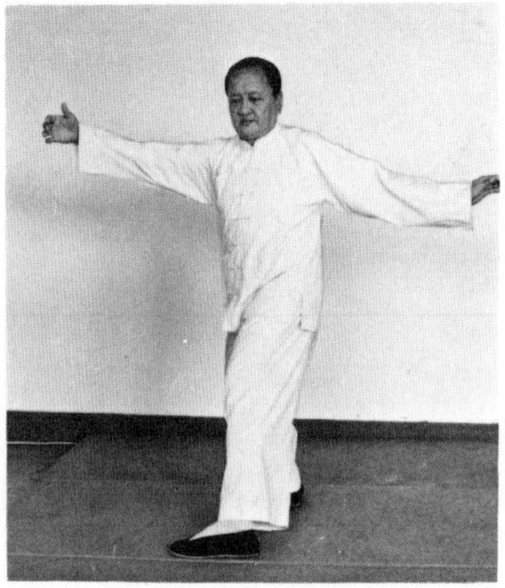

FIG. 16-6B ·

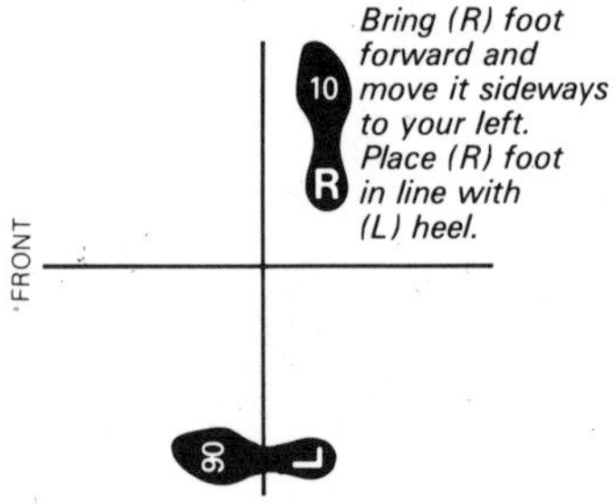

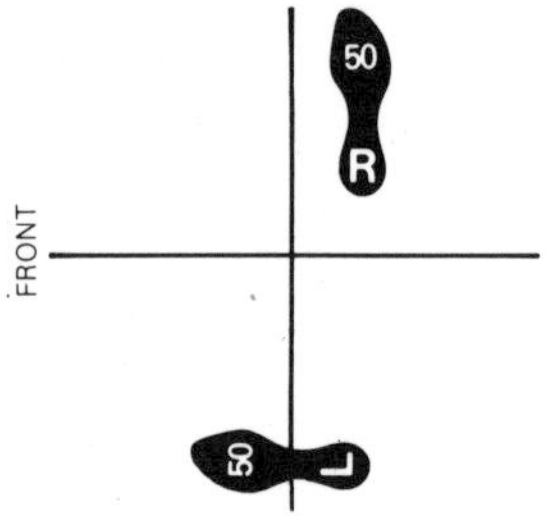

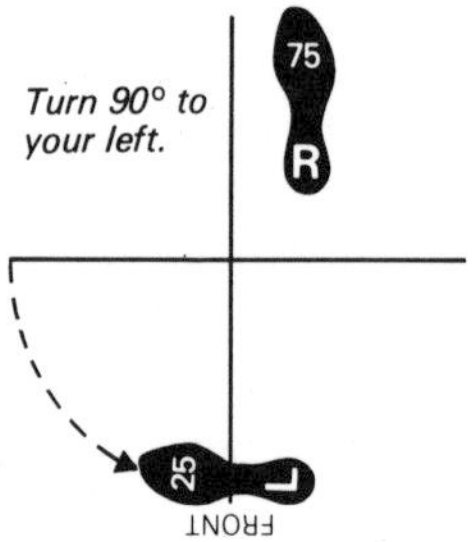

Bring (R) foot forward and move it sideways to your left. Place (R) foot in line with (L) heel.

10

R

FRONT

90 L

Gradually shift weight to (R) foot.

50

R

FRONT

50 L

Turn 90° to your left.

75

R

25 L

FRONT

Zhǒu dǐ kàn chuí

Punch under elbow

Continue moving forward until nearly all your weight is on your front **(L) foot.** Then lift **(R) foot** off the ground and bring it forward until (R) toes lie beside (L) heel. Move **(R) foot** sideways, as far to your right as possible, while keeping nearly all your weight on the **(L) foot.** Place **(R) foot** down so it is in line with and perpendicular to (L) foot (Fig. 16-4). When you have placed the **(R) foot** flat on the ground, gradually shift weight from (L) to **(R) foot.** This can be done by straightening the (L) leg. Maintain the same height by bending the **(R) knee.** Throughout both these moves you have moved neither arms nor body (Fig. 16-5).

When approximately 75 per cent of your weight is on the **(R) foot,** turn **waist** 90° to your left. Pull in **(L) hip** in order to execute this turn properly. Keep both arms fixed in relation to your body so that they would each also have traversed through 90° (Fig. 16-6).

Zhǒu dǐ kàn chuí

Punch under elbow

The last part involves mainly the movement of your hands. First adduct **(L) shoulder** and, keeping **(L) elbow** extended, let (L) arm fall to your side. Coordinate this with turning **body** and head 45° to your right (Fig. 16–7).

Continue the move by lifting **(L) heel** off the ground and shifting entire weight onto **(R) foot**. Now abduct **(L) shoulder** to lift (L) arm away from your body. When (L) upper arm is level with (L) shoulder, flex **(L) elbow** to raise (L) forearm to an upright position. The (L) arm would now have described a semicircle. Your **(L) palm** will be facing you at this point. You should, simultaneously, turn your **body** another 45° to your right (Fig. 16–8).

Finally, flex **(R) elbow** to bring (R) hand beneath (L) elbow. Clench **(R) hand** into a fist with the row of knuckles vertical. Rotate **(L) wrist** so (L) palm now faces your right with the narrow edge of the (L) hand facing forward. At the same time, move **(L) leg** to your right till it is in line with (R) heel. Place only **(L) heel** on the ground and do not put any weight on it (Fig. 16–9). An important point to note in executing this move is that you should maintain a constant height throughout, particularly when the (L) arm is describing its arc.

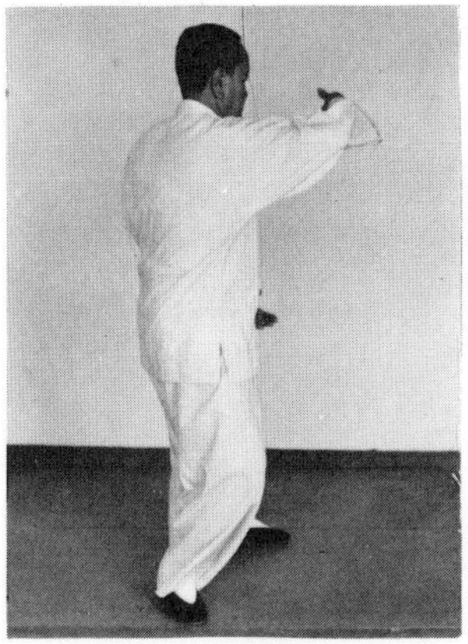

FIG. 16-7F

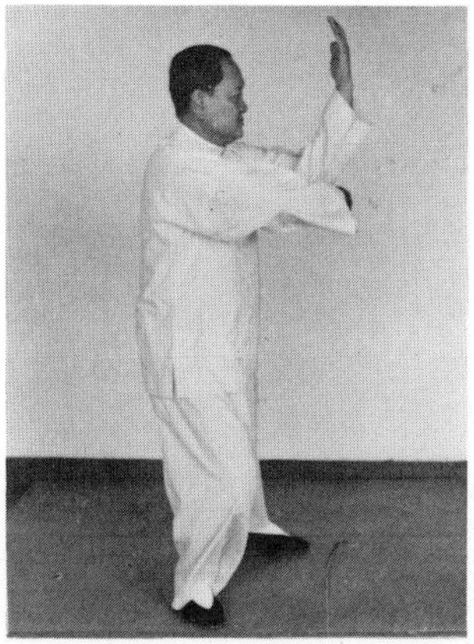

FIG. 16-8F

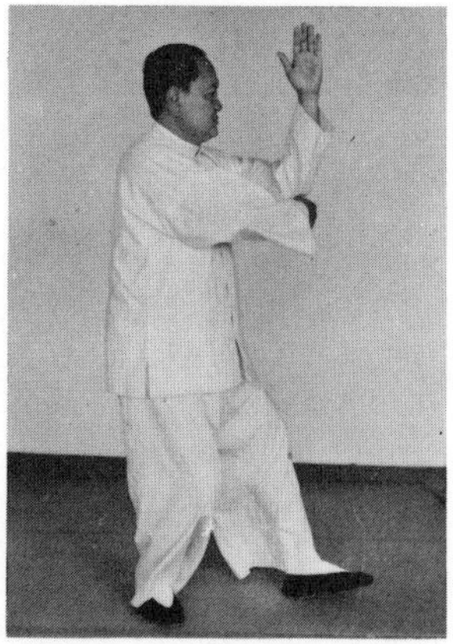

FIG. 16-9F

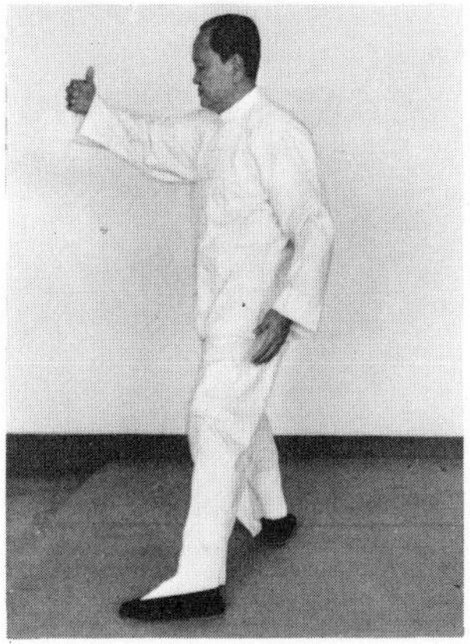

FIG. 16-7B

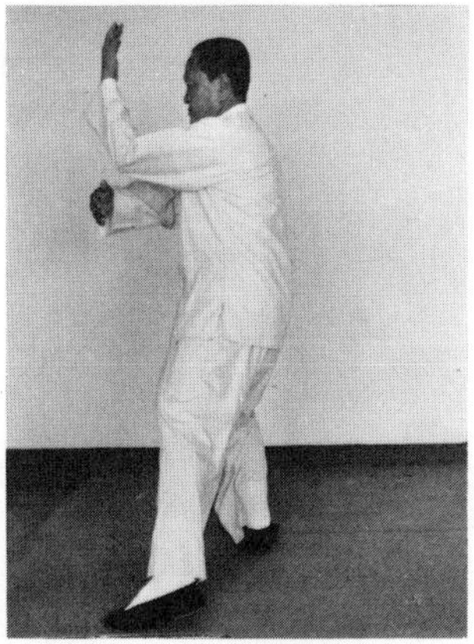

FIG. 16-8B

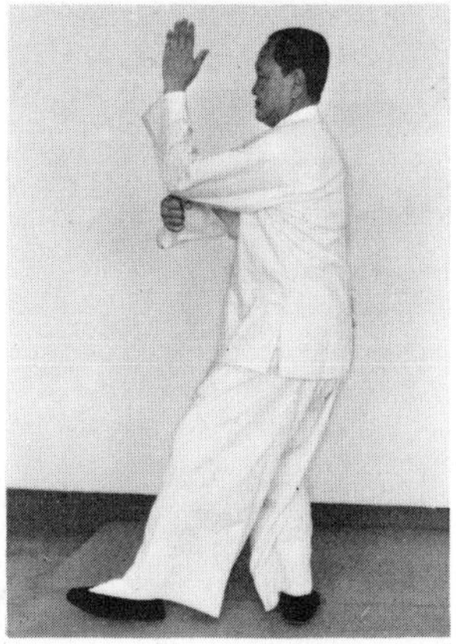

FIG. 16-9B

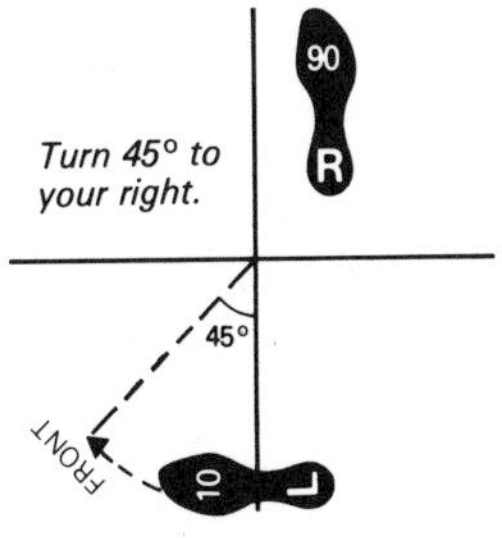

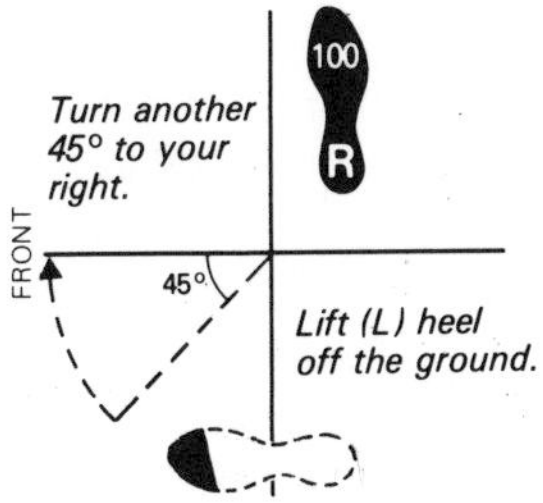

Turn 45° to your right.

Turn another 45° to your right.

Lift (L) heel off the ground.

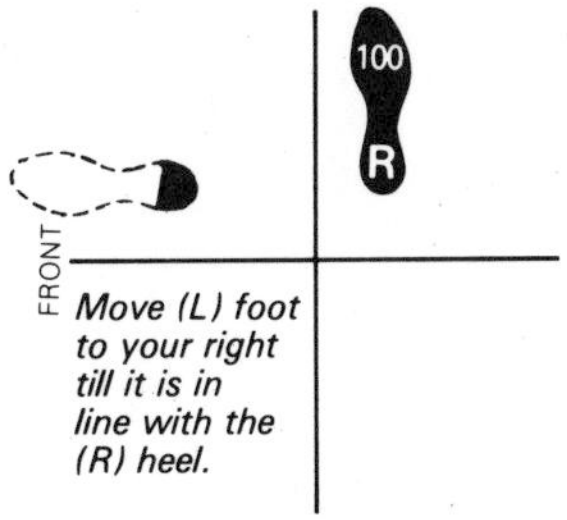

Move (L) foot to your right till it is in line with the (R) heel.

Keep weight on (R) foot.

55

倒撵猴

Dào niǎn hóu

Step back and repulse monkey

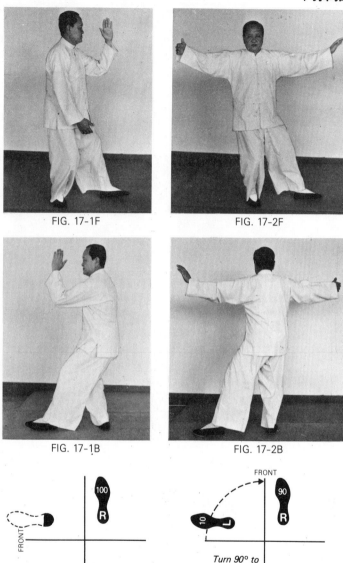

FIG. 17-1F

FIG. 17-2F

FIG. 17-1B

FIG. 17-2B

FRONT

100
R

FRONT

Turn 90° to your right.

FRONT

90
R

10
L

This involves a series of five repetitive movements that enable you to retreat in an orderly manner. This is a particularly important move, and its repetition helps ensure sufficient practice.

The first two moves, illustrated here, involve movements of your hands and waist only. Initially adduct **(R) shoulder** then extend **(R) elbow** so (R) arm can fall to your side. Do not move either (L) arm (which should be perpendicular to the ground) or body (Fig. 17–1).

Now turn **body** 90° to your right. As you do this stretch out **both arms** till they are in line with each other and parallel to the ground. You can do this by abducting the **(R) shoulder** and keeping **(R) elbow** fully extended. Extension of the **(L) elbow** will also allow you to stretch out (L) arm fully. Note that your head should follow the turn of your body so it now faces the same direction (Fig. 17-2). Throughout both moves, remember to keep weight focused on (R) foot.

Keep weight on back (R) foot.

Dào niǎn hóu

Step back and repulse monkey

倒撵猴

Flex **(R) elbow** to pull in (R) forearm with palm facing (R) ear. Turn **body** 45° to your left. Rotate **(L) wrist** so (L) palm now faces you. Keep eyes focused on (L) palm and weight on back **(R) foot** (Fig. 17–3).

Now move **(L) foot** straight back and place it down, heel first. Make sure toes point forward and heel is in line with toes. Both feet are now at right angles to each other (Fig. 17–4).

Next straighten (R) leg to transfer weight onto back **(L) foot.** As you do this, move both arms in tandem. Bring (L) arm to your side by adducting **(L) shoulder.** As (L) arm falls, rotate then abduct **(R) shoulder** so (R) arm is brought forward. Do not exert any tension on (R) forearm. Rotate **(R) wrist** so (R) palm faces forward. Coordinate this movement so that as one arm is pulled in, the other is pushed forward. As you complete this move, turn your **body** another 45° to your left and permit **(R) foot** to turn 90° so both feet now face forward (Fig. 17–5).

Next turn **waist** 90° to your left. As you do this, abduct **(L) shoulder** while keeping (L) elbow fully extended, to raise (L) arm till it is at shoulder level and parallel to the ground. Extend **(R) elbow** to stretch out (R) arm fully (Fig. 17–6).

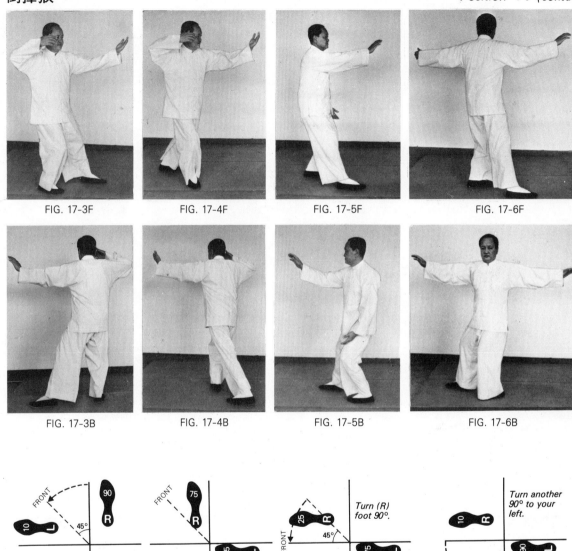

FIG. 17-3F   FIG. 17-4F   FIG. 17-5F   FIG. 17-6F

FIG. 17-3B   FIG. 17-4B   FIG. 17-5B   FIG. 17-6B

Turn 45° to your left.

Move (L) foot straight back.

Turn (R) foot 90°.

Turn another 45° to your left.

Turn another 90° to your left.

Move (L) leg back then transfer weight to (L) foot.

倒攆猴

Dào niǎn hóu
Step back and repulse monkey

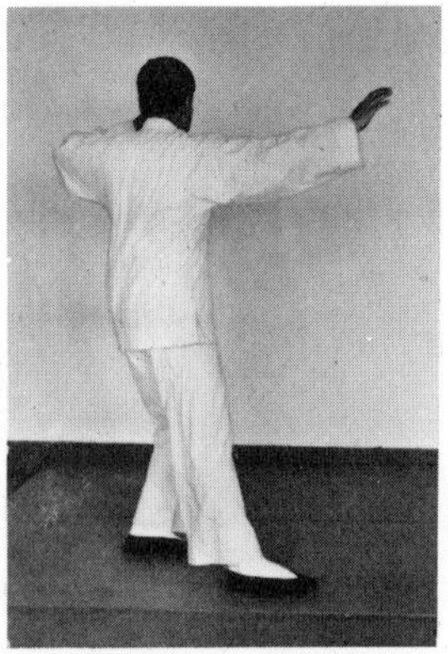

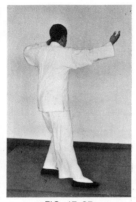

FIG. 17-7F

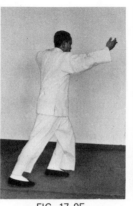

FIG. 17-8F

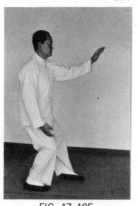

FIG. 17-9F

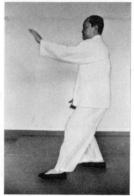

FIG. 17-10F

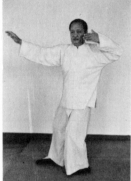

FIG. 17-7B

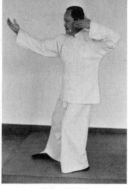

FIG. 17-8B

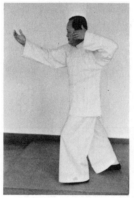

FIG. 17-9B

FIG. 17-10B

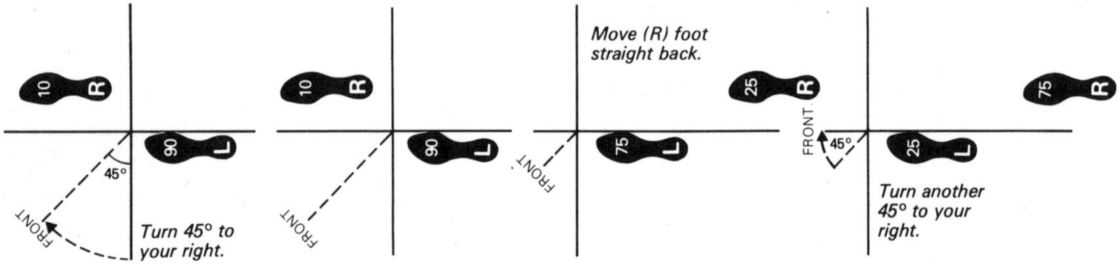

This series of pictures illustrate the continuation of the move, with one major difference – you now turn your body in the opposite direction.

This time flex **(L) elbow** and pull (L) forearm toward you with palm facing (L) ear. Turn **body** 45° to your right. Rotate **(R) wrist** so the (R) palm now faces you. Keep eyes focused on (R) palm and weight on back **(L) foot.** Both feet should be parallel to each other and pointing forward (Figs. 17–7 and 17–8).

Now move **(R) foot** back as far as possible and place it down, heel first. Make sure that both the toes and heel point forward and both feet are parallel to each other (Fig. 17–9). Begin shifting your weight back onto **(R) foot** and, as you do this, move both arms in tandem. Bring **(R) arm** to the side by adducting **(R) shoulder,** while lifting (L) arm by first rotating and then abducting **(L) shoulder.** Remember to first rotate **(L) shoulder** so that the (L) elbow is turned till it points downward. Coordinate the movements of your arms so that as one is pulled in, the other is pushed forward and it appears that both arms are linked with an invisible string (Fig. 17–10).

Turn 45° to your right.

Move (R) foot straight back.

Turn another 45° to your right.

Move (R) leg back then shift weight onto (R) foot.

Dào niǎn hóu

Step back and repulse monkey

The same set of moves is repeated three more times – the third and fifth sets being identical to the first set (Figs. 17–2 to 17–5) and the fourth set being identical to the second (Figs. 17–6 to 17–10). The third set is illustrated here. You should conclude this set with **(R) foot** in front and most of your weight concentrated on back **(L) foot** (Fig. 17–14).

A few of the more important points to note in executing these moves are:

1 Your feet should move back in a straight line with toes and heels aligned and pointing straight forward.

2 Do not exert any strength in the forearm when you thrust it forward. Ensure that it is relaxed with elbow held well below the palm. Concentrate the thrust on the elbow to stretch shoulder joint.

3 Try to keep an even height throughout, particularly when you move back. Avoid bobbing up and down as this would dissipate energy and make practice a waste of time.

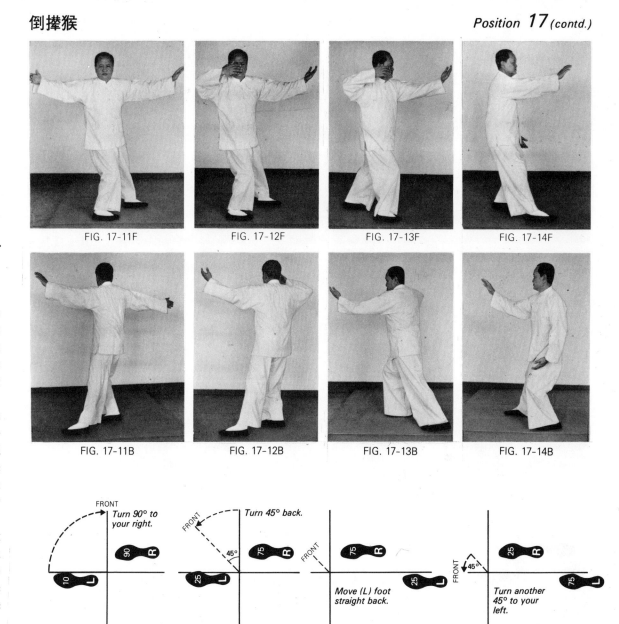

FIG. 17-11F   FIG. 17-12F   FIG. 17-13F   FIG. 17-14F

FIG. 17-11B   FIG. 17-12B   FIG. 17-13B   FIG. 17-14B

FRONT
Turn 90° to your right.

Turn 45° back.

Move (L) foot straight back.

Turn another 45° to your left.

Move (L) foot back then transfer weight onto it.

斜飞势

Xié fēi shì

Diagonal flying

This move is illustrated in six photographs. The first three, shown on this page, involve mainly the transfer of weight from one leg to another.

First adduct **(R) shoulder** and, keeping **(R) elbow** extended, let (R) arm fall across your body with (R) palm facing the centre of the body (Fig. 18–1). Then flex **(L) elbow** to lift (L) forearm up through an angle of 45°. Remember to keep at least 75 per cent of your weight on the **(L) foot** (Fig. 18–2).

Holding arms in position, lift **(R) foot** off the ground and pull it inward, toward the (L) foot. Allow (R) toes to touch the ground lightly and do not exert any weight on it. Extend **(L) wrist** to straighten (L) hand. Note that the open **(L) palm** faces the same direction as the (R) leg. Rotate **(R) shoulder** so (R) arm is held slightly away from your body (Fig. 18–3).

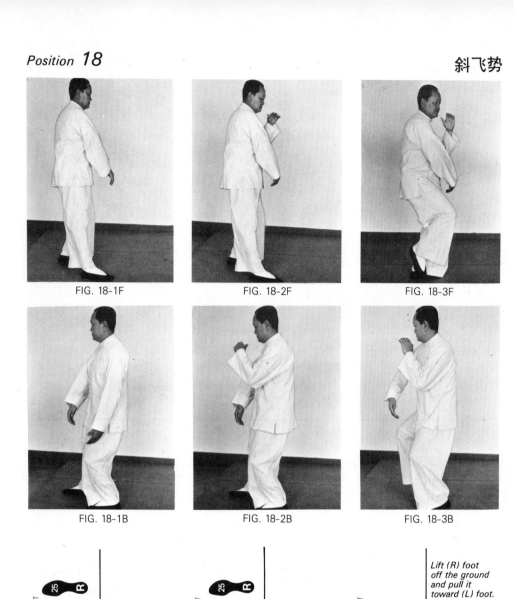

FIG. 18-1F   FIG. 18-2F   FIG. 18-3F

FIG. 18-1B   FIG. 18-2B   FIG. 18-3B

FRONT 25 R 75 L

FRONT 25 R 75 L

FRONT Lift (R) foot off the ground and pull it toward (L) foot. 100 L

Concentrate weight on (L) foot.

Xié fēi shì
Diagonal flying

斜飞势

Step out and move **(R) foot** to your right. Place it at an angle of 135° to the (L) foot. Note that both heels are still in line with each other though your feet point in different directions. Follow this movement with your **body** turning 45° to your right. Notice how Chia quite clearly keeps most of his weight on his back **(L) foot** at this stage (Fig. 18–4).

Gradually shift your weight from back (L) foot to front **(R) foot.** Do this by straightening **(L) foot.** At the same time allow (L) arm to fall to your side by extending (L) elbow. Abduct **(R) shoulder** to lift (R) upper arm upward and to your right. Make sure it describes this semicircle within the range of the (L) arm (Fig. 18–5).

Complete the movement by turning body another 90° to your right. You will now face the same direction as your (R) foot. Straighten **(L) leg** and turn **(L) foot** 45° to your right. This will shift most of your weight to your **(R) foot.** Rotate **(R) shoulder** to let (R) arm complete its sweep so (R) elbow lies directly over (R) knee. The **(R) hand** should be at eye level and **(R) palm** facing you. At this point (R) knee, hip and elbow should be in line with (R) toes, (L) arm should lie by your side, and **(L) palm** should face the floor (Fig. 18–6).

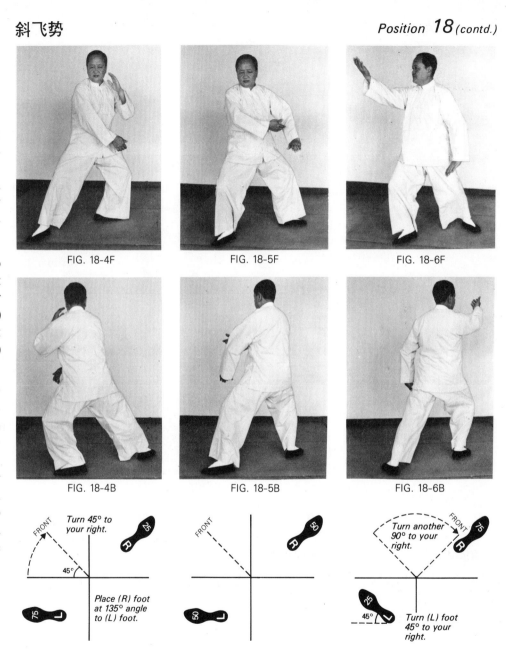

FIG. 18-4F   FIG. 18-5F   FIG. 18-6F

FIG. 18-4B   FIG. 18-5B   FIG. 18-6B

Turn 45° to your right.   *Place (R) foot at 135° angle to (L) foot.*

Turn another 90° to your right.   *Turn (L) foot 45° to your right.*

Gradually shift weight to (R) foot.

云手

Yún shǒu
Wave hands in clouds

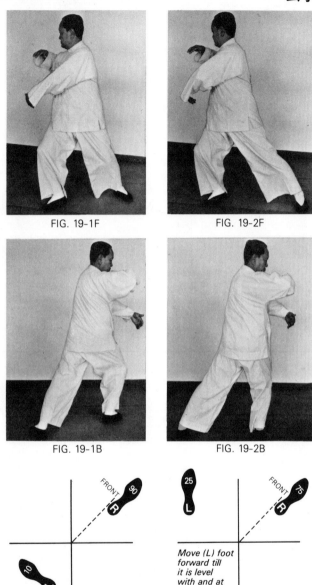

FIG. 19-1F

FIG. 19-2F

FIG. 19-1B

FIG. 19-2B

Move (L) foot forward till it is level with and at a 45° angle to the (R) foot.

Keep weight on (R) foot.

This is another series of repetitive moves. In this instance the move is repeated seven times. The emphasis of this series of moves is on the turning of your waist. If performed well, this will form one of the main sources of your strength.

The photographs here illustrate how you would get into position to begin. First move forward, transferring nearly all your weight onto front **(R) foot.** In this position, rotate **(L) wrist** and flex **(L) elbow** to bring in (L) forearm with (L) palm facing you. At the same time rotate **(R) wrist** so (R) palm faces downward, then flex (R) elbow to bring (R) forearm down till it is parallel to the ground. At this point, (L) arm is below the right with both palms facing each other (Fig. 19–1).

Keeping most of your weight on front **(R) foot,** move **(L) leg** forward. Place it down at the same level as (R) foot, making sure (L) toes point straight forward. Notice that (R) foot is pointing at an angle of 45° away from (L) foot (Fig. 19–2). Keep eyes focused on (R) hand throughout.

Yún shǒu

Wave hands in clouds

The next three moves together make up the first of the seven repetitive parts of *yún shǒu*.

Initially, turn **body** another 45° to your right and then allow (R) arm to fall to your side by adducting **(R) shoulder,** then extending **(R) elbow.** This downward movement of the (R) arm should take place as you raise the **(L) arm** so, as it falls, (R) arm moves on the outside of (L) arm. Keep **(L) elbow** flexed and adduct (L) shoulder so (L) forearm is perpendicular to (L) upper arm and both are parallel to the ground (Fig. 19–3).

Now turn **body** 180° to your left. Keep both arms still and in front of you as you turn. In this process transfer your weight from (R) to **(L) foot** by straightening (R) leg and pulling in (L) hip. Allow **(R) foot** to turn 45° to the left so it is now parallel to (L) foot and points straight forward (Fig. 19–4).

When you are in this position, turn **(L) wrist** so (L) palm now faces downward. Adduct **(L) shoulder** and extend **(L) elbow** to let (L) arm drop to your side. Keeping **(R) elbow** flexed, raise **(R) arm** till it is parallel to the ground with its palm facing you. This interchange of arm positions brings them back to their starting positions, only this time you are facing the opposite direction (Fig. 19–5).

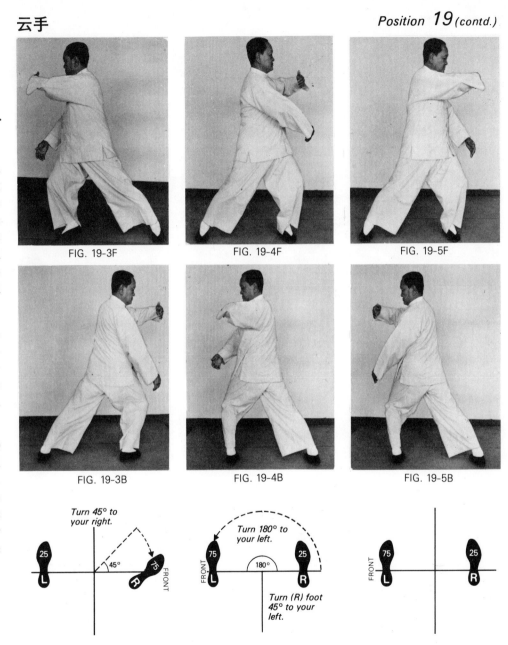

FIG. 19-3F FIG. 19-4F FIG. 19-5F

FIG. 19-3B FIG. 19-4B FIG. 19-5B

Turn 45° to your right.

Turn 180° to your left.

Turn (R) foot 45° to your left.

Transfer weight to (L) foot.

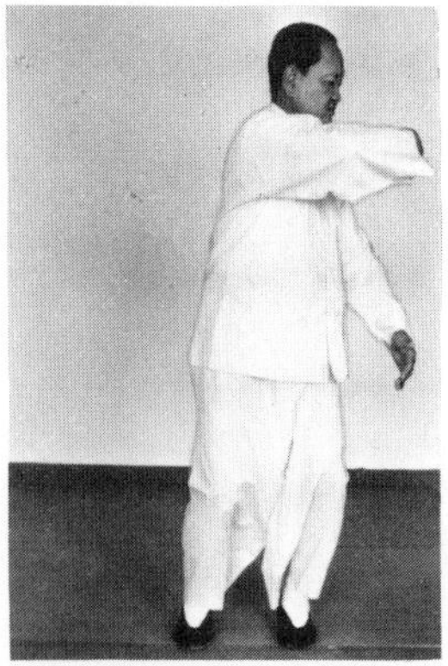

云手

FIG. 19-6F

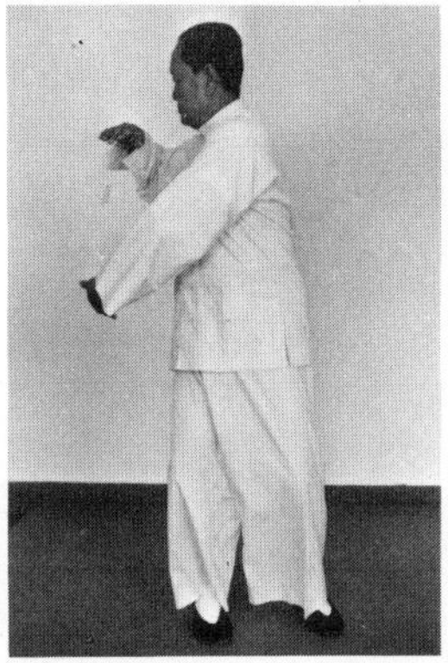

FIG. 19-7F

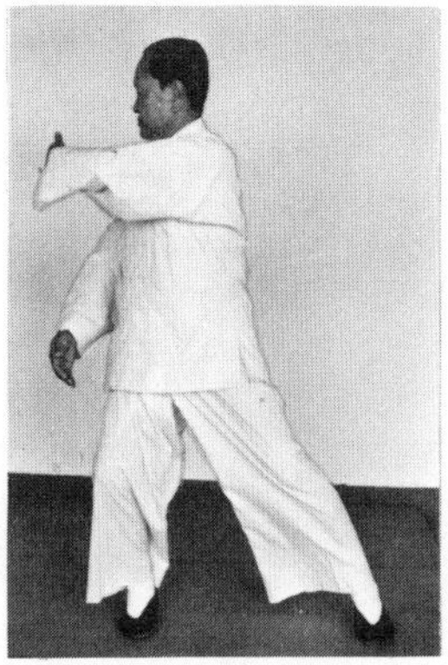

FIG. 19-8F

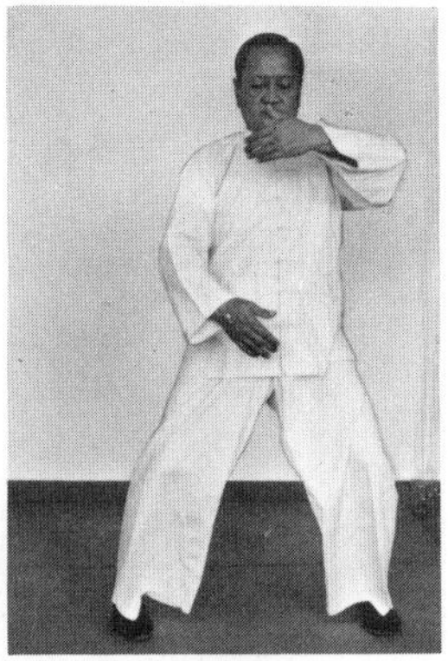

FIG. 19-9F

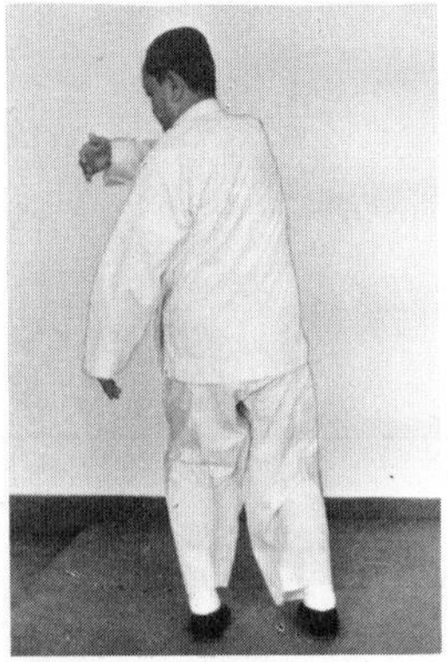

FIG. 19-6B

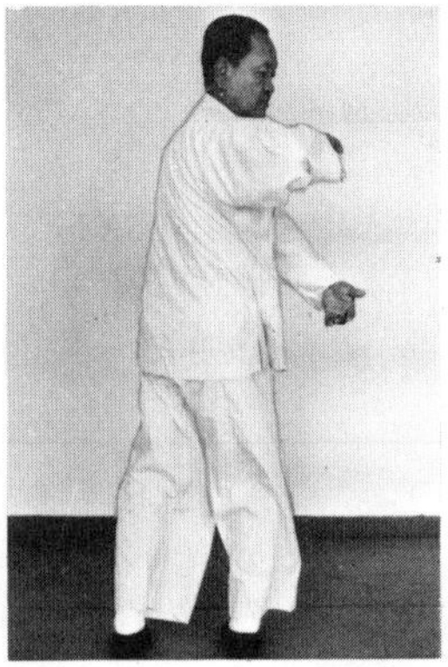

FIG. 19-7B

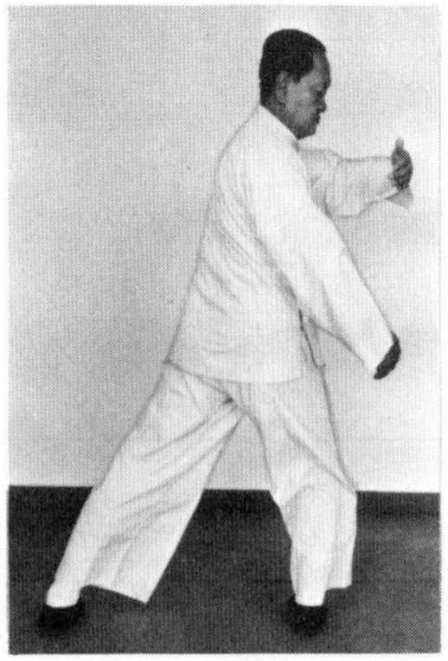

FIG. 19-8B

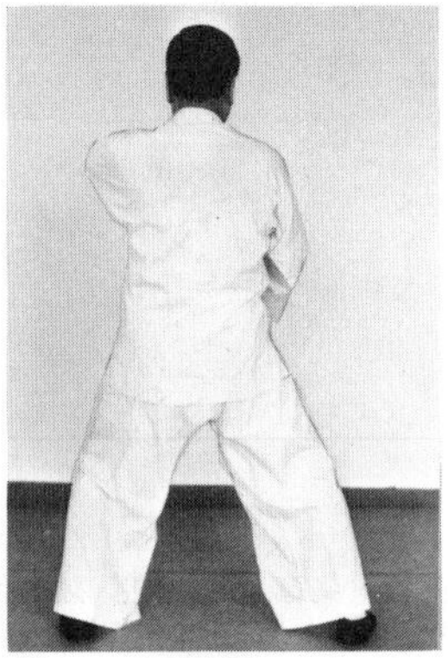

FIG. 19-9B

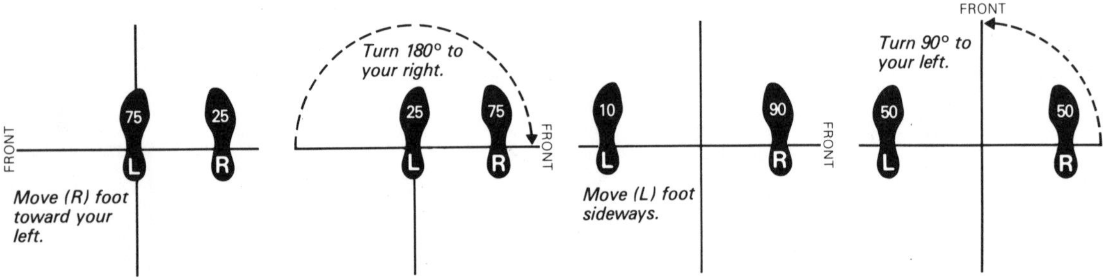

Yún shǒu

Wave hands in clouds

Figs. 19–6 and 19–7 together illustrate the second of the seven repetitive parts of *yún shǒu*. Initially, move **(R) foot** sideways to your left. Place it on the same level as (L) foot, keeping your weight mostly on the **(L) foot** (Fig. 19–6). Next turn **waist** 180° to your right, simultaneously shifting weight to **(R) foot.** Bend both knees slightly as you turn to keep height level throughout this move. Note that you do not move your arms at this point (Fig. 19–7).

Keeping most of your weight on the **(R) foot** and with body maintaining its direction, move **(L) foot** sideways and place it parallel to the (R) foot. Repeat interchange of arm positions by letting **(R) arm** fall to your side and simultaneously raising **(L) arm.** Remember that the higher arm always falls to the outside of the rising lower arm (Fig. 19–8). Then gradually turn **waist** to your left, initially through 90° (Fig. 19–9) and then through another 90° (Fig. 19–10). In this move the turn is made at the waist. The arms remain stationary in relation to body and move only together with it.

FRONT

75 25

FRONT

Move (R) foot toward your left.

Turn 180° to your right.

25 75

FRONT

10 90

FRONT

Move (L) foot sideways.

Turn 90° to your left.

FRONT

50 50

Initially transfer weight to (R) foot. Then move (L) foot sideways to your left and gradually shift weight to it.

Yún shǒu

Wave hands in clouds

Fig. 19–10 illustrates the completion of the third part of *yún shǒu*. Notice that whenever you complete a turn to your left, you would have completed on odd number of turns, say three or five. A turn to your right would always mark the completion of an even-numbered turn. This will help you remember the number of repetitive moves that you have made.

Figs 19–11 to 19–13 illustrate the fourth turn – to your right. It begins with an interchange in **arm** positions, with the right arm being brought above the left (Fig. 19–11), followed by the movement of the **(R) foot** toward the left (Fig. 19–12) and finally the turning of your **waist**, initially through 45° and then another 135° to the right. This should be accompanied by the concomitant weight transfer to the **(R) foot** (Fig. 19–13). You are now facing the direction in which you began the move.

云手

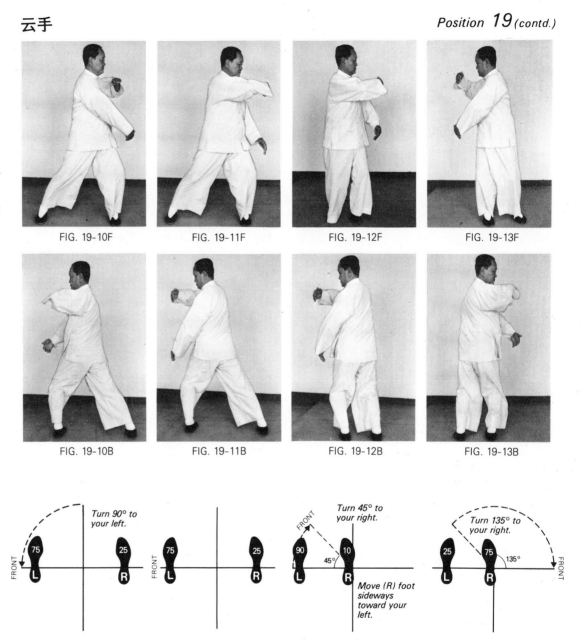

FIG. 19-10F FIG. 19-11F FIG. 19-12F FIG. 19-13F

FIG. 19-10B FIG. 19-11B FIG. 19-12B FIG. 19-13B

Turn 90° to your left.

Turn 45° to your right.

Move (R) foot sideways toward your left.

Turn 135° to your right.

Complete transfer of weight to (L) foot. Then move (R) foot toward your left and shift weight to it.

云手

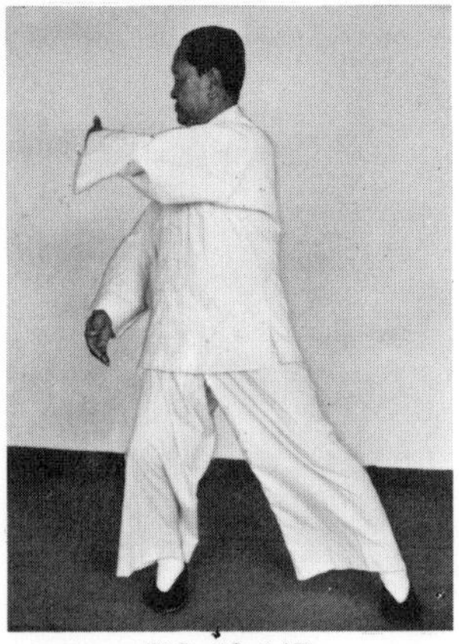

FIG. 19-14F

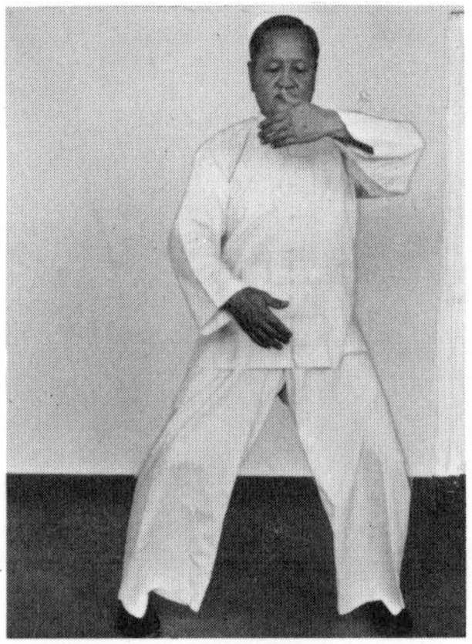

FIG. 19-15F

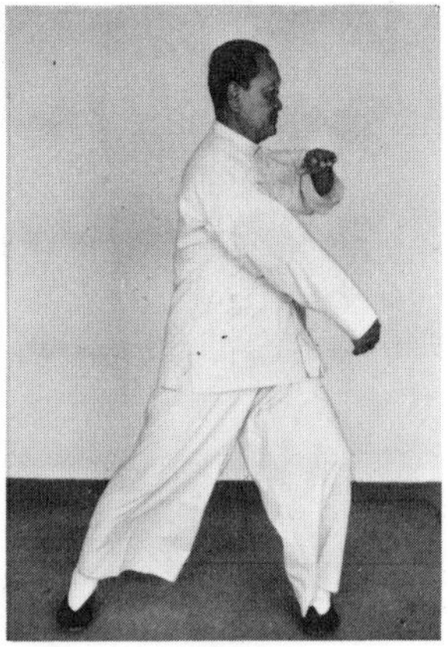

FIG. 19-16F

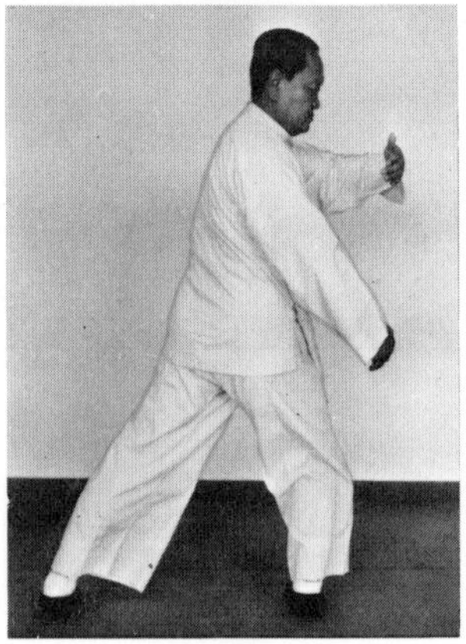

FIG. 19-14B

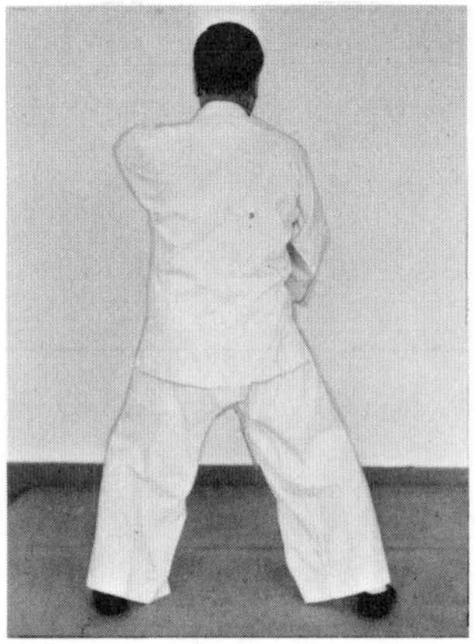

FIG. 19-15B

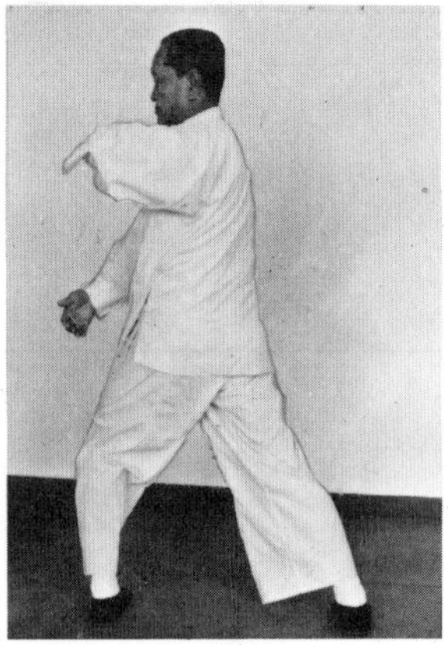

FIG. 19-16B

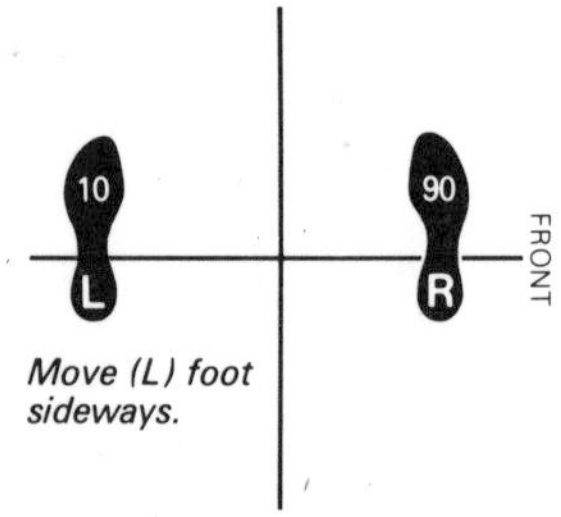

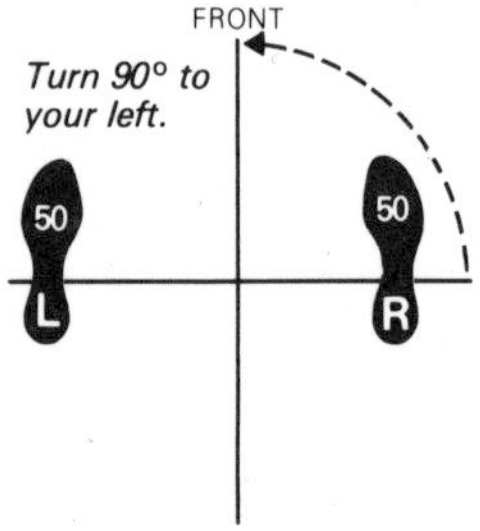

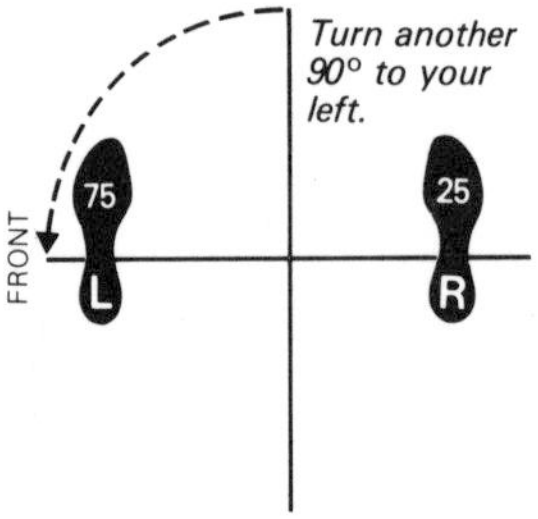

Yún shǒu
Wave hands in clouds

The pictures (Figs. 19–14 to 19–16) show Chia demonstrating the fifth part of *yún shǒu*. The moves involved are exactly similar to the third part (Figs. 19–8 to 19–10). Two more parts, the sixth and seventh, are required to complete this particular movement. These are not illustrated as they are similar to others that have been described. The sixth move is a repetition of the move shown in Figs. 19–5 to 19–7 and again in Figs. 19–11 to 19–13. The seventh move was previously illustrated in Figs. 19–8 to 19–10 and here in Figs. 19–14 to 19–16. The completion of the seventh move will bring you to the position illustrated in Fíg. 19–16.

A few of the more important points to keep in mind as you execute these moves are:

1 Your waist, not head or hands, is involved in the turns from left to right and back again.

2 Keep eyes on the palm of the hand that is in front of you (the higher one). This will help you to synchronise the turning of head with body.

3 Keep knees slightly bent as you turn as this will enable you to maintain a constant height and to transfer weight efficiently from one foot to the other.

Move (L) foot sideways.

Turn 90° to your left.

Turn another 90° to your left.

Move (L) foot sideways then transfer weight to it.

Dān biān

Single whip

This move rounds off Chapter Two. From your position at the end of the last move, adduct **(L) shoulder** then extend (L) elbow to let (L) arm fall to your side. Keep most of your weight on the **(L) foot** (Fig. 20–1).

Next move **(R) foot** straight forward, making sure it still points forward when you place it down. Move neither hands nor body which is now facing 90° away from the (R) foot. Keep most of your weight concentrated on **(L) foot** (Fig. 20–2).

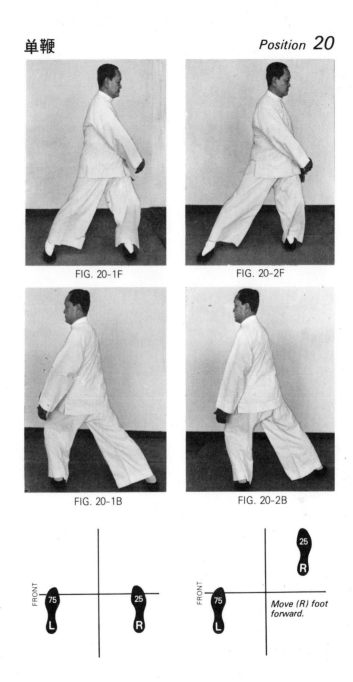

FIG. 20-1F

FIG. 20-2F

FIG. 20-1B

FIG. 20-2B

Move (R) foot forward.

Keep weight on (L) foot.

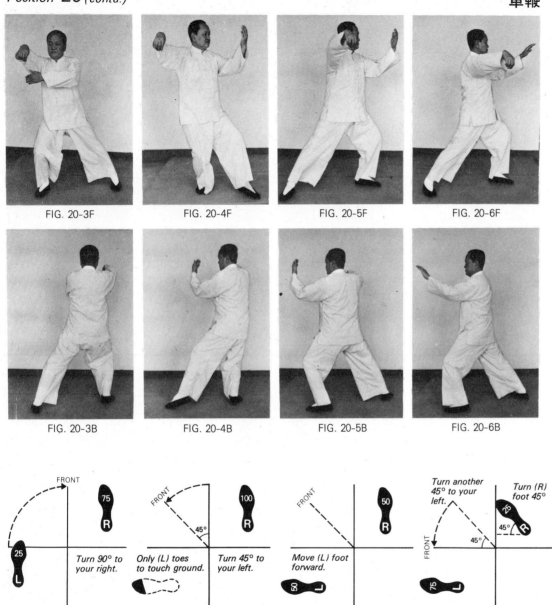

FIG. 20-3F　　FIG. 20-4F　　FIG. 20-5F　　FIG. 20-6F

FIG. 20-3B　　FIG. 20-4B　　FIG. 20-5B　　FIG. 20-6B

Initially move weight to (R) foot. Then pivot on (L) toes, step out and transfer bulk of weight to (L) foot.

Dān biān

Single whip

Now turn **body** 90° to your right so you now face the direction (R) foot is pointing. Transfer your weight to **(R) foot** and simultaneously abduct **(R) shoulder** to lift (R) arm forward. At this point, flex **(R) wrist** and simultaneously abduct (L) shoulder to raise (L) arm. Flex **(L) elbow** to bring (L) palm below (R) elbow (Fig. 20–3).

Complete *dān biān* by carrying out the moves illustrated from Figs. 20–4 to 20–6. These have been described earlier for Position 5 (pages 28–30). In order to achieve this classic posture you have to keep your body straight. Often when you attempt to do this you will find that the sole of your (R) foot tends to be lifted off the ground. One way to prevent this is to keep (R) knee slightly bent and pointing in the same direction as (R) toes. Remember to keep only a fraction of your weight on the (R) foot.

This is the end of the second chapter. You have now progressed halfway through the basic course. At this point, review the first two parts of the exercise until you are reasonably familiar with the sequence of movements before progressing further. It would probably take you about one or two months to come to this stage if you have been practising regularly and mastering about one or two positions each week.

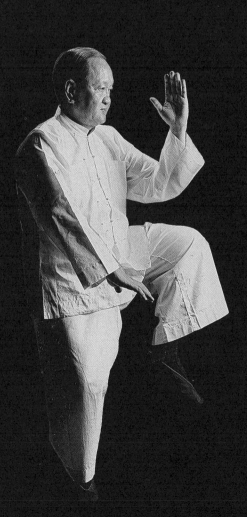

Chapter Three

This part of the exercise consists of eleven moves of which eight are new and the remaining three are moves that you have learnt before. Technically, this and the last part of the exercise are the most difficult to master – appropriately so for as you get more conversant with the exercise, more complex moves can be introduced with less difficulty. Chapter Three begins with Position 21, *xìa shì*, and ends at Position 31, *dān biān*.

下势

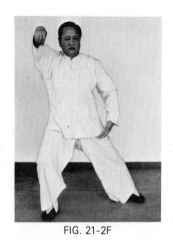

FIG. 21-1F

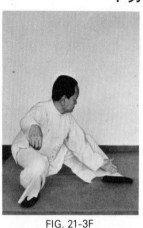

FIG. 21-2F

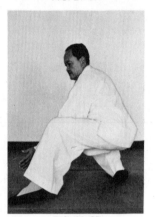

FIG. 21-3F

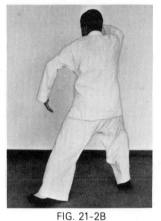

FIG. 21-1B

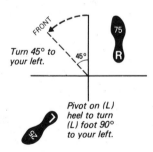

FIG. 21-2B

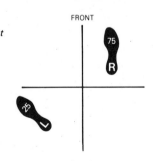

FIG. 21-3B

Xià shì

Squatting single whip

Turn **(R) foot** 45° to your right and, while maintaining the same height, turn **body** 90° in the same direction. Allow **(L) foot** to turn 45° also and at the same time straighten (L) leg to transfer most of your weight onto **(R) foot**. Keep **(R) hand** extended with **(R) wrist** flexed. Flex **(L) elbow,** pulling (L) forearm toward you. Note that **(L) palm** is open and faces you (Fig. 21-1).

Now adduct **(L) shoulder** to bring (L) arm, sideways, to your side. Do not move and keep your weight concentrated on the (R) leg (Fig. 21-2).

Finally squat on **(R) leg** and turn **body** 45° to your left. Keep **(L) arm** close to the inner side of (L) leg. Next pivot on **(L) heel** to turn (L) foot 90° to your left. Keep (R) arm outstretched and (R) wrist flexed (Fig. 21-3).

FRONT

Turn 90° to your right.

Turn (R) foot 45° to your right.

75

R

45°

25

L

45°

Turn (L) foot 45° to your right.

FRONT

75

R

25

L

FRONT

Turn 45° to your left.

75

R

45°

25

L

Pivot on (L) heel to turn (L) foot 90° to your left.

Shift weight to (R) foot.

Jīn jī dú lì (zuǒ shì)

Golden cock stands on one leg, left

Basically, this consists of four movements that allow you to move forward, upward and finally to lift (R) leg at the hip.

From your previous squatting position, move forward and upward, keeping **(L) shoulder** abducted and **elbow** fully extended to raise (L) arm from beside (L) leg up to eye level. Keep **(L) palm** open and make sure it faces you. As you move upward, turn both **body** and **(R) foot** 45° to your left. At the same time, straighten (R) leg to transfer weight to front **(L) foot** (Fig. 22–1).

Next lift **(R) heel** so only (R) toes remain in contact with the ground. All your weight should now be on front **(L) foot.** At the same time, turn **(L) wrist** 90° so (L) palm faces downward. Adduct **(R) shoulder** to bring (R) arm toward you, making sure it is relaxed with (R) palm facing upward (Fig. 22–2).

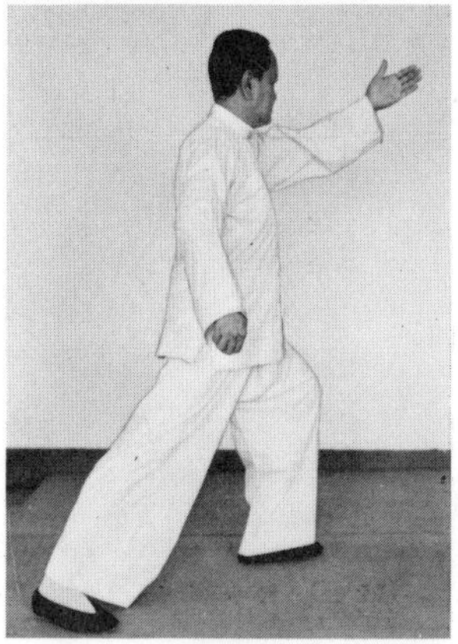

FIG. 22-1F

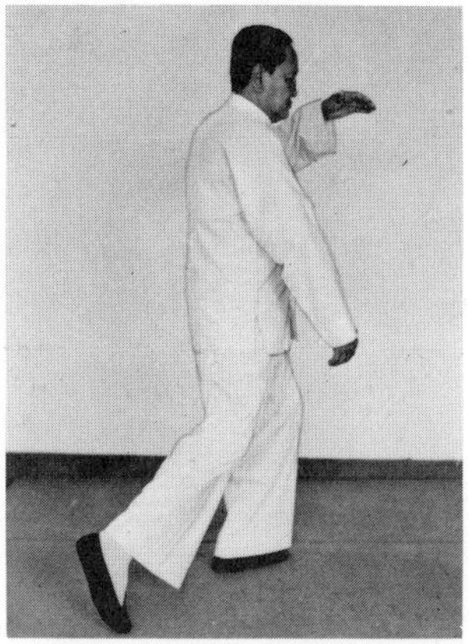

FIG. 22-2F

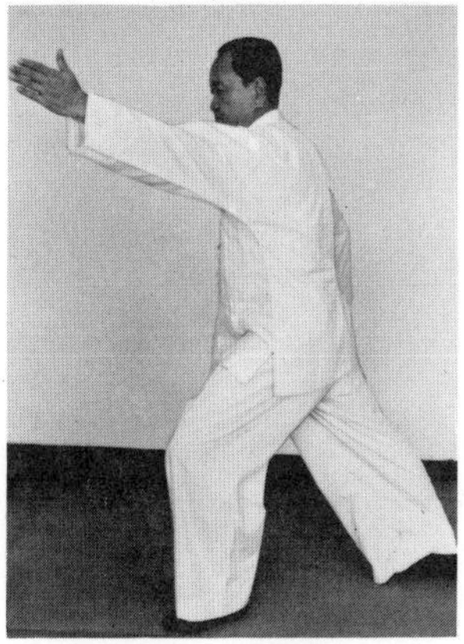

FIG. 22-1B

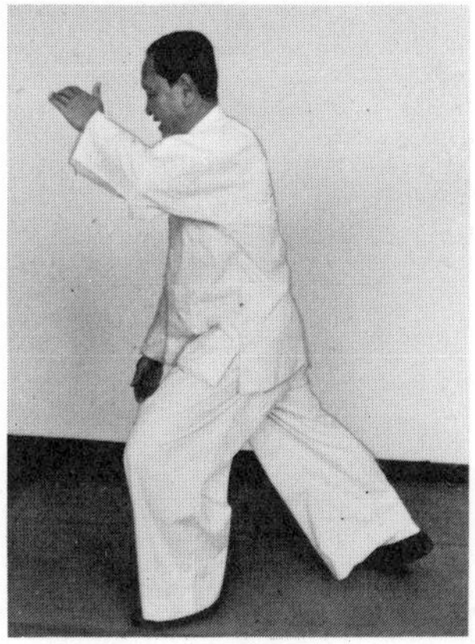

FIG. 22-2B

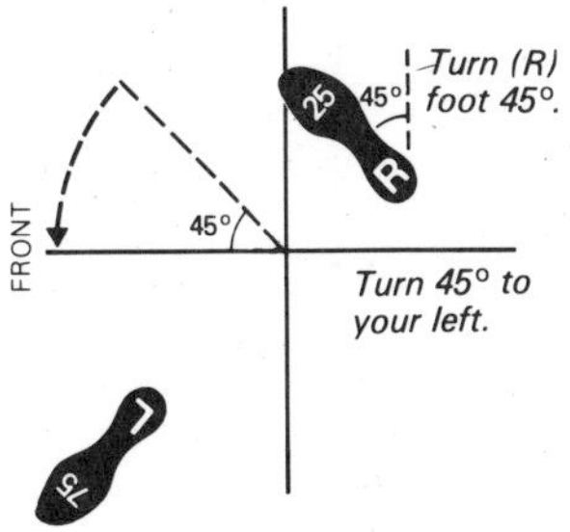

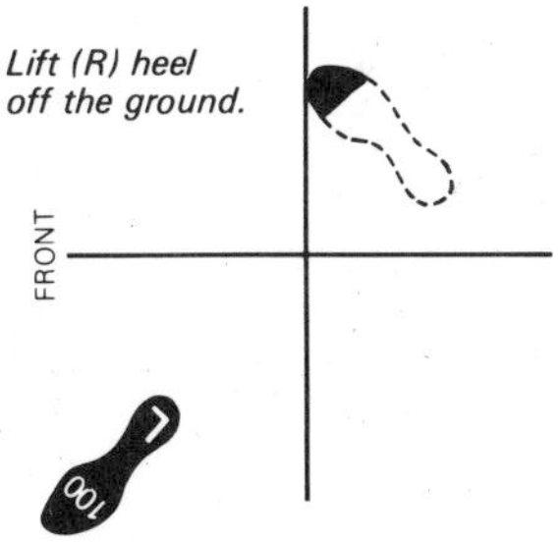

Turn (R) foot 45°.

Turn 45° to your left.

Lift (R) heel off the ground.

Move upward and forward. Put weight onto front (L) foot.

71

金鸡独立（左式）

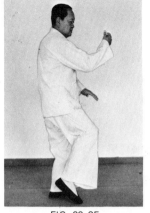

FIG. 22-3F

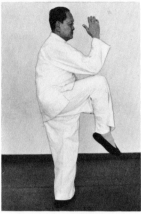

FIG. 22-4F

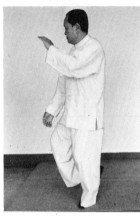

FIG. 22-3B

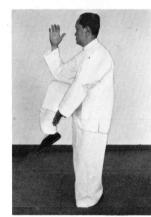

FIG. 22-4B

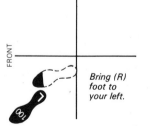

Bring (R) foot to your left.

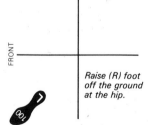

Raise (R) foot off the ground at the hip.

Concentrate weight on (L) foot.

Jīn jī dú lì (zuǒ shì)

Golden cock stands on one leg, left

Bring **(R) leg** forward up to (L) foot and permit only (R) toes to touch the ground. Keep all your weight on **(L) foot.** Do not turn body or move arms at this stage (Fig. 22–3).

Adduct **(R) hip** to raise (R) leg, keeping thigh parallel to the floor with **(R) ankle** extended to point toes. This will keep (R) shin perpendicular to (R) thigh. Your weight would, of course, still be concentrated on the **(L) foot.** As you raise your leg, simultaneously abduct **(R) shoulder** to raise (R) arm. Then flex **(R) elbow** and rotate **(R) wrist** so (R) forearm is upright with the narrow edge of (R) palm facing forward. Your (R) palm now faces left. Place **(R) elbow** on (R) knee. Extend and spread **(R) fingers,** keeping them upright and separated from each other.

As you raise the (R) foot, adduct **(L) shoulder** and extend (L) elbow to lower (L) arm. Movement of arms should be made in conjunction with each other – lower (L) arm at the same rate at which you raise (R) arm. This will help you maintain your balance. At the end of the move, the **(L) arm** should be slightly bent and held at a slight angle away from your body. Try to make these moves as slowly as possible and remember to keep **(L) knee** slightly bent in order to maintain the same height throughout (Fig. 22–4).

Jīn jī dú lì (yòu shì)

Golden cock stands on one leg, right

This is a repetition of the last move, except that you now stand on the (R) instead of on the (L) foot.

First bring **(R) leg** down and place (R) foot behind and perpendicular to (L) foot. Concentrate weight on front **(L) foot** and do not move either arm (Fig. 23–1).

Now, keeping your arm still, straighten front **(L) leg** and move backward to shift weight onto back **(R) foot.** Bend **(R) knee** slightly to remain level. Keep as straight a posture as possible and look straight ahead (Fig. 23–2).

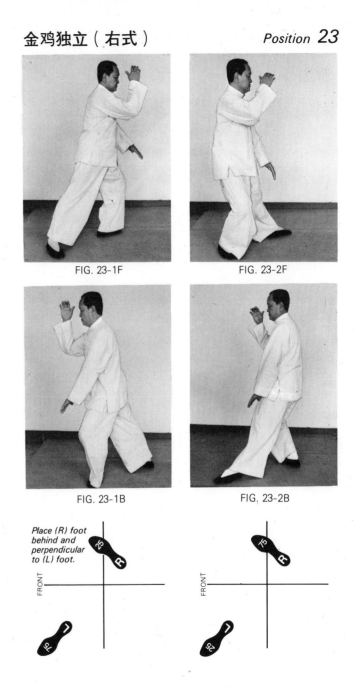

FIG. 23-1F

FIG. 23-2F

FIG. 23-1B

FIG. 23-2B

Place (R) foot behind and perpendicular to (L) foot.

Shift weight to back (R) foot.

金鸡独立（右式）

Jīn jī dú lì (yòu shì)
Golden cock stands on one leg, right

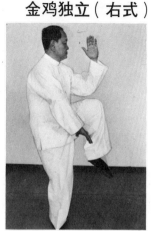

FIG. 23-3F

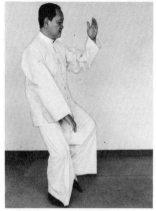

FIG. 23-4F

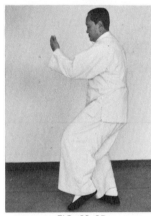

FIG. 23-3B

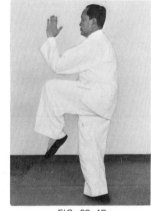

FIG. 23-4B

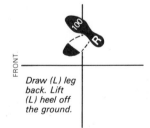

Draw (L) leg back. Lift (L) heel off the ground.

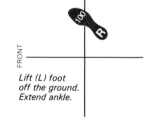

Lift (L) foot off the ground. Extend ankle.

Keep weight on back (R) foot.

When all your weight is on the back **(R) foot,** pull **(L) foot** back then lift **(L) heel** off the ground. At the same time adduct **(R) shoulder** then extend **(R) elbow** to let (R) arm fall to your side. Adduct **(L) shoulder,** raise (L) arm and flex (L) elbow so (L) forearm is now in an upright position (Fig. 23-3).

Finally adduct **(L) hip** to lift (L) leg till knee is in line with (L) hip. Extend **(L) ankle** to point toes. The (L) shin will now be perpendicular to the (L) thigh and to the ground. Keep **(R) knee** slightly bent. Place **(L) elbow** lightly on top of (L) knee and turn **(L) wrist** 90° so the narrow edge of (L) hand faces forward and (L) palm faces right. The (R) arm should be held by the side of your body, slightly outward with the hand forward at the (R) knee. **(R) palm** faces downward at this point. Extend **(R) fingers** so they lie apart from each other and are not curled up (Fig. 23-4).

Yòu fēn jiǎo

Separate right foot

右分脚

This intricate move is illustrated over a series of ten frames, Figs. 24–1 to 24–10. It involves carrying out a low kick with the (R) foot and a hit with the (R) hand. The move becomes difficult to carry out when you are required to perform it slowly and in a relaxed manner.

Initially, extend **(L) elbow** until (L) forearm is parallel to the ground with (L) palm facing upward. Maintaining your position, i.e. with **(L) foot** off the ground, abduct **(R) shoulder** and lift (R) elbow until it is in line with the (L) elbow. At this point, flex **(R) elbow** and pull (R) forearm toward you. Continue this movement until **(R) palm** is above and faces (L) elbow (Fig. 24–1).

Now, while holding arms in position, bring **(L) foot** down and place it behind and perpendicular to (R) foot. Place it as far back as you can while maintaining at least 75 per cent of your weight on front (R) foot (Fig. 24–2).

Next flex **(L) elbow** and pull in (L) forearm toward you till it is below (R) elbow. Notice the **(L) palm** now faces your body. At the same time extend **(R) elbow** so (R) forearm is now upright with edge of (R) palm facing forward. Simultaneously, turn **body** 45° to your right while keeping most of your weight on front **(R) foot** throughout (Fig. 24–3).

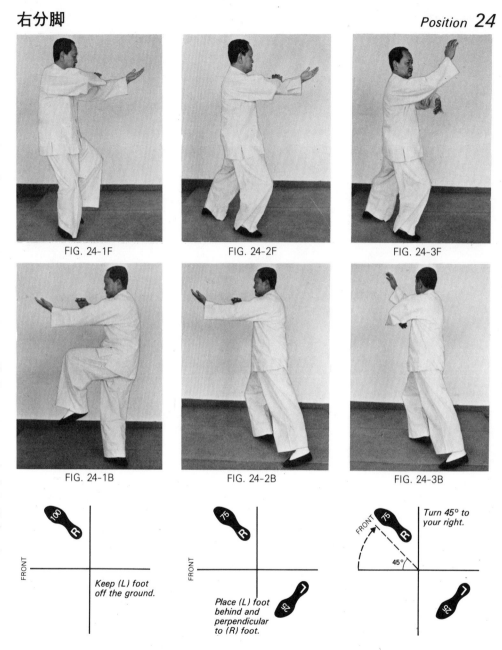

FIG. 24-1F   FIG. 24-2F   FIG. 24-3F

FIG. 24-1B   FIG. 24-2B   FIG. 24-3B

Keep (L) foot off the ground.

Place (L) foot behind and perpendicular to (R) foot.

Turn 45° to your right.

Keep weight on (R) foot.

右分脚

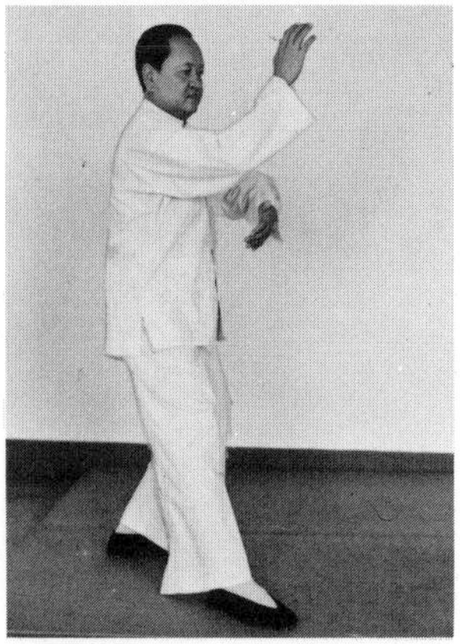

FIG. 24-4F

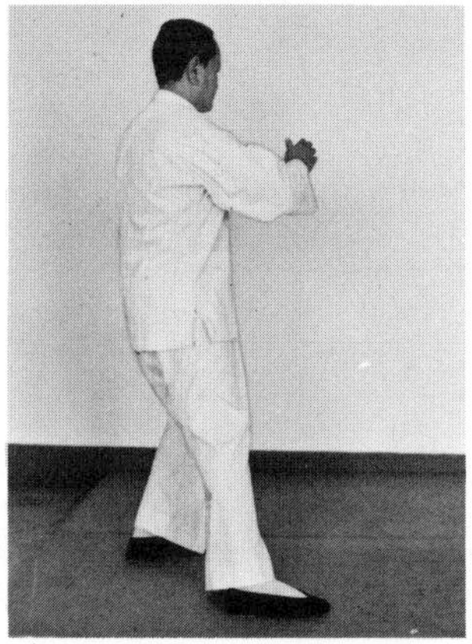

FIG. 24-5F

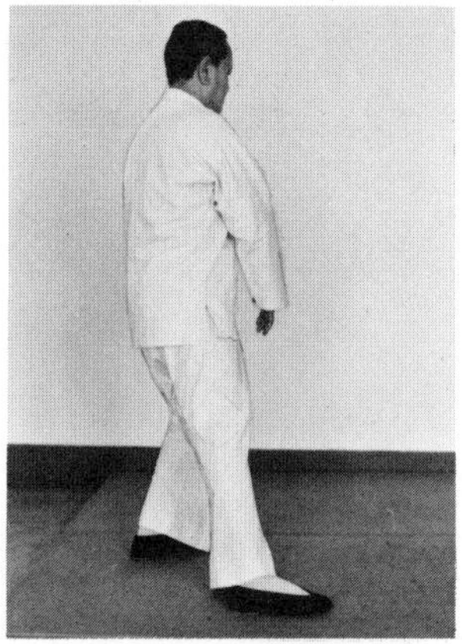

FIG. 24-6F

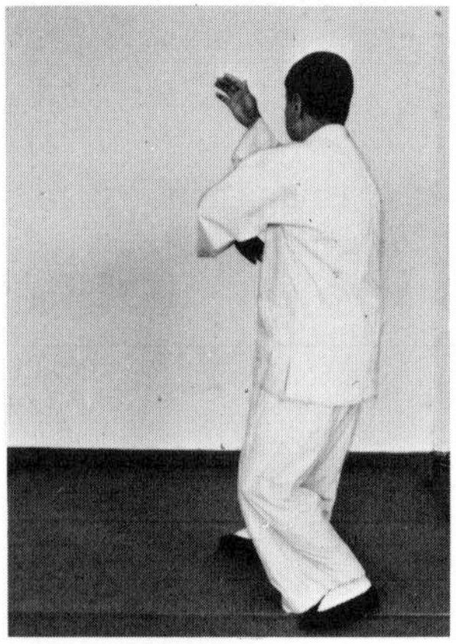

FIG. 24-4B

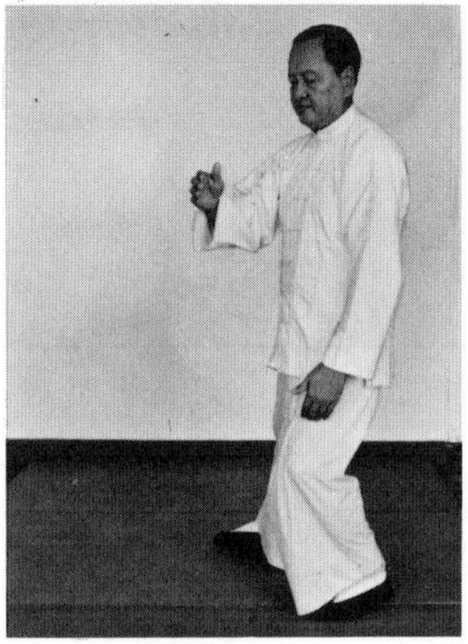

FIG. 24-5B

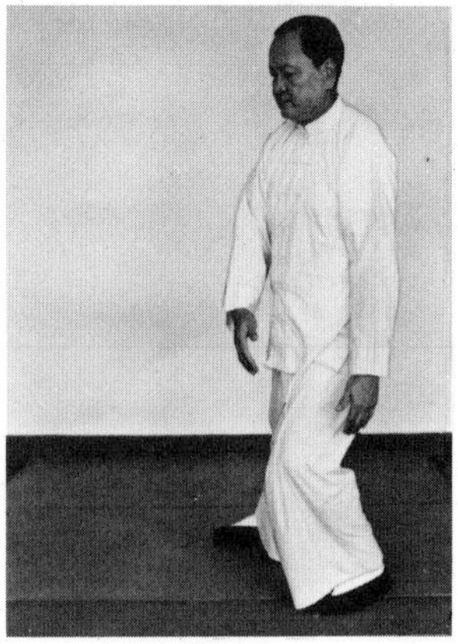

FIG. 24-6B

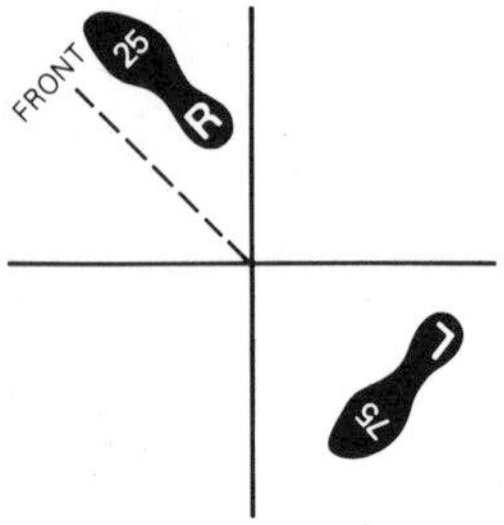

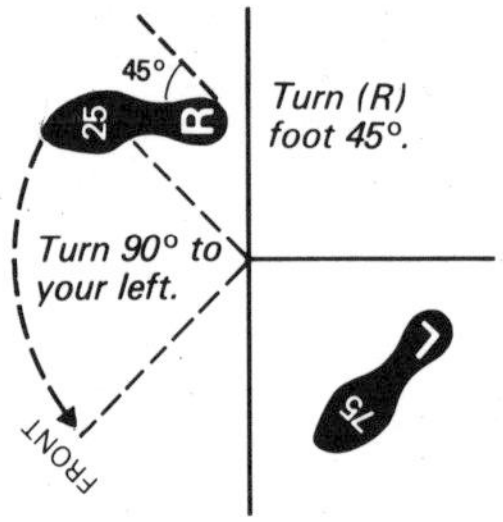

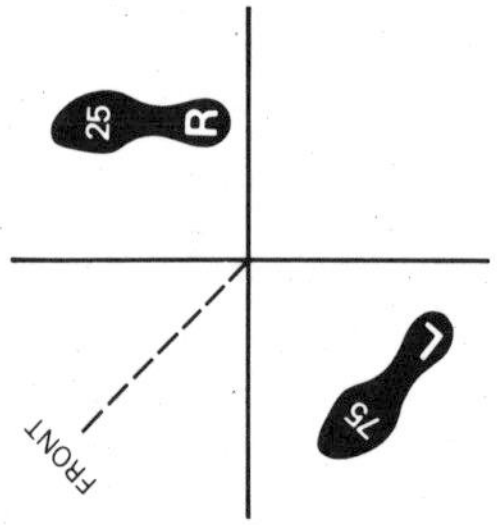

Yòu fēn jiǎo

Separate right foot

Keeping arms in position, straighten front (R) leg and move back to put at least 75 per cent of your weight on back **(L) foot.** When you carry out this move, ensure that the **(L) knee** is bent with the kneecap pointing to the toes (Fig. 24-4).

Next turn **body** 90° to your left. The **(R) foot** should turn 45° in the same direction. While turning, adduct **(L) shoulder** and then extend **(L) elbow** to allow (L) arm to fall by your side. At the same time, adduct **(R) shoulder** to let (R) forearm fall toward your left (Fig. 24-5).

When your arms are completely relaxed, allow your weight to sink down to back **(L) foot.** This can be achieved if you relax and stretch the (L) shoulder and (L) elbow as much as possible. Both palms should face inward. Notice that even though Chia is relaxed, he still extends his **fingers** so that they are straight and separated from each other (Fig. 24-6).

FRONT — 25 — R — 75

45°
25 — R
Turn (R) foot 45°.
Turn 90° to your left.
FRONT — 75

25 — R
FRONT — 75

Transfer weight to back (L) foot and keep it there.

Yòu fēn jiǎo

Separate right foot

In the same position, abduct **(L) shoulder** to raise (L) arm. Then flex **(L) elbow** to bring (L) forearm in till it is at right angles to (L) upper arm. The **(L) palm** should face you at this point (Fig. 24–7).

Next abduct **(R) shoulder** to raise (R) arm forward till **(R) wrist** is in contact with and below (L) wrist. Both hands should be kept open with both palms facing you. At the same time, lift **(R) heel** off the ground and transfer all your weight to **(L) foot** (Fig. 24–8).

Upon completing the last move, turn **body** 90° to your right. Simultaneously, pivot on **(R) toes** to enable you to pull in (R) hip. As you swivel to your right, abduct both **shoulders** to raise both arms laterally. Rotate both **wrists** so open palms now face away from you. The **(R) palm** should be furthest from you as it was originally held below the (L) palm (Fig. 24–9).

Finally, pull **(L) shoulder** back and move (L) arm backward. At the same time extend **(R) elbow** so (R) forearm falls forward with the narrow edge of (R) hand pointing downward. You should, as you move your arms, simultaneously extend **(R) knee** and **ankle** till (R) shin is in line with (R) thigh. Do not exert any force at (R) hip. This kick should take place very gently with the **(R) foot** only a few centimetres off the floor. Try not to straighten the (L) leg as you execute this move (Fig. 24–10).

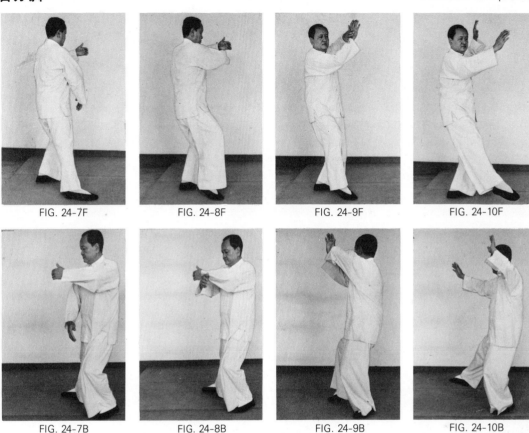

FIG. 24-7F   FIG. 24-8F   FIG. 24-9F   FIG. 24-10F

FIG. 24-7B   FIG. 24-8B   FIG. 24-9B   FIG. 24-10B

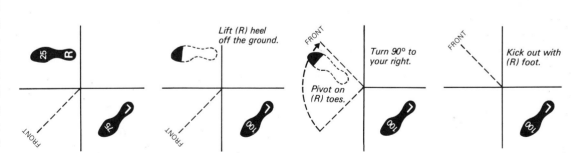

Keep weight on back (L) foot.

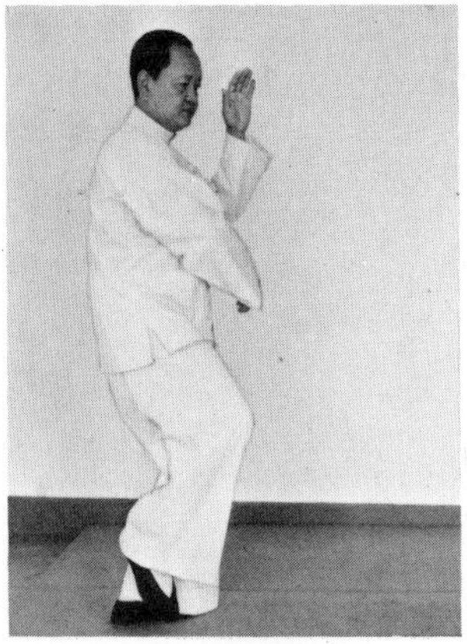

FIG. 25-1F

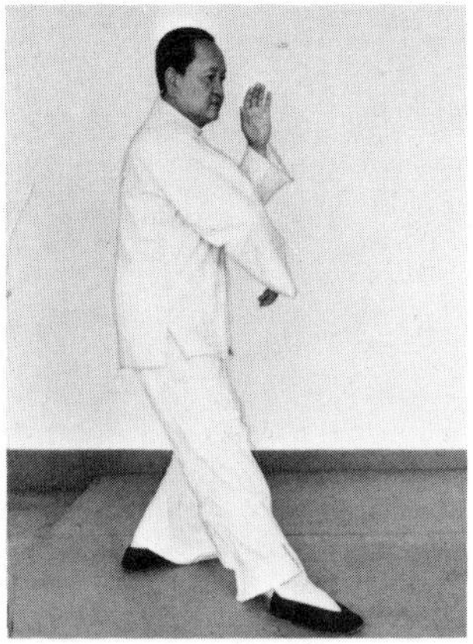

FIG. 25-2F

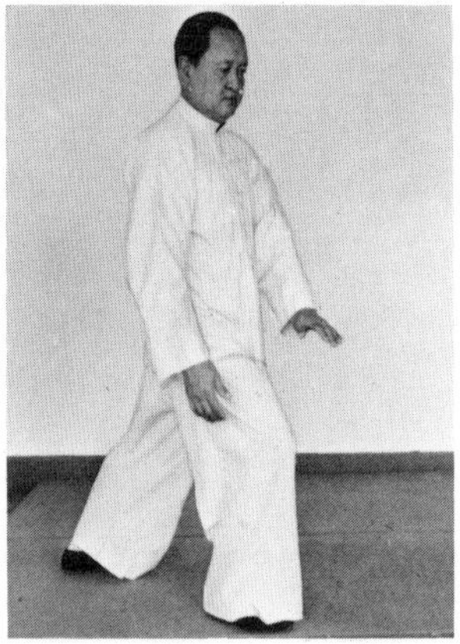

FIG. 25-3F

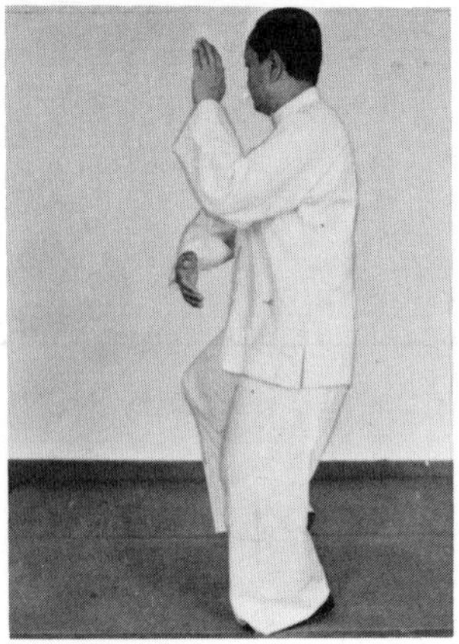

FIG. 25-1B

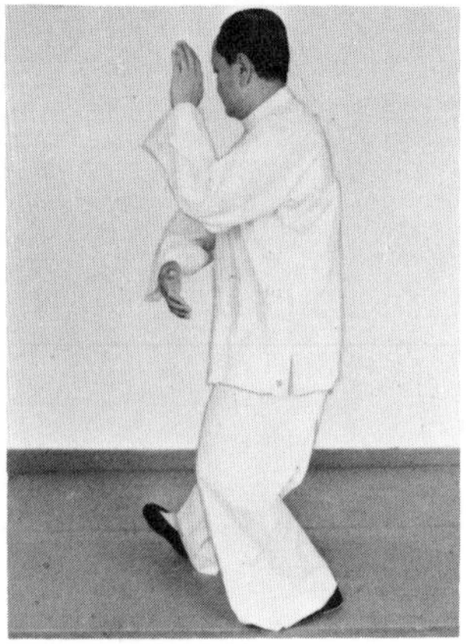

FIG. 25-2B

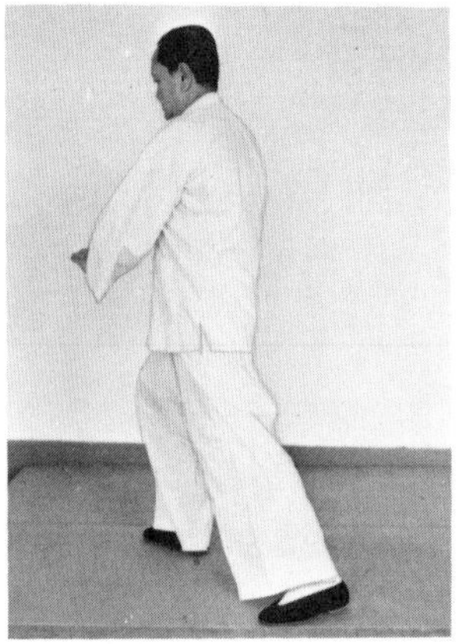

FIG. 25-3B

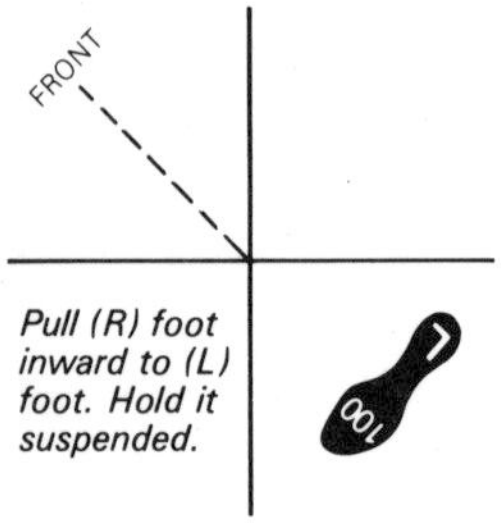

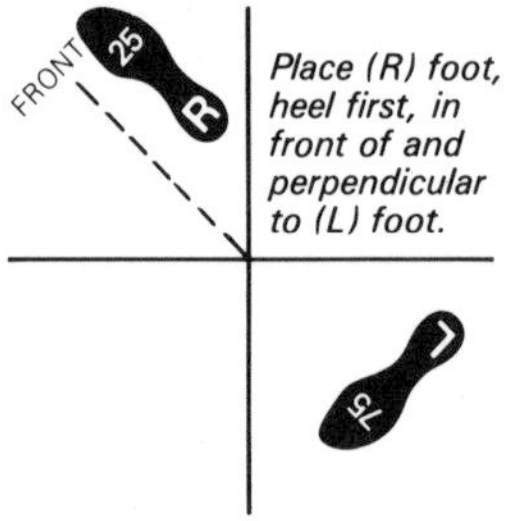

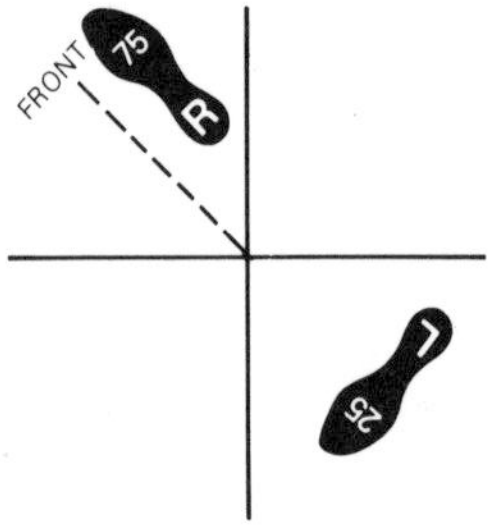

Pull (R) foot inward to (L) foot. Hold it suspended.

Place (R) foot, heel first, in front of and perpendicular to (L) foot.

Zuǒ fēn jiǎo
Separate left foot

This is essentially a repetition of the previous move except that the (L) foot – and not the right – kicks out, at a different angle. This not only enables you to practise the move, in combat it teaches you how to elude an attack and how to counter-attack from a different angle.

Initially, pull back all the limbs which were extended at the end of the last move. Adduct **(L) shoulder** and allow (L) elbow to sink downward to your side, with **(L) forearm** still upright. At the same time flex **(R) elbow** so (R) forearm is pulled across your body with open palm facing you. Finally flex **(R) knee** to pull in (R) shin so it is held suspended near the (L) foot (Fig. 25–1).

Next, while keeping weight on back **(L) foot,** extend **(R) knee** and place (R) foot down. Place it, heel first, forward and perpendicular to (L) foot (Fig. 25–2).

Now move forward, transferring your weight onto front **(R) foot** by extending **(L) knee** and straightening (L) leg. As you carry this out, extend both **elbows** to permit both arms to fall on either side (Fig. 25–3).

Transfer weight to front (R) foot.

Zuǒ fēn jiǎo

Separate left foot

The next four moves are exactly the same as those shown earlier (page 77), except that you now rest on your (R) foot and kick out with your left. It is also executed at a 90° angle away from the first set of moves.

Initially, abduct **(R) shoulder** to raise (R) arm. Then flex **(R) elbow** to bring (R) forearm to a position perpendicular to (R) upper arm (Fig. 25-4). Abduct **(L) shoulder** and bring up **(L) arm** until both wrists cross each other with the narrow edge of both hands facing downward. At the same time lift **(L) heel** off the ground and move **(L) leg** to your right until (L) toes are in line with (R) heel. This sequence of leg movements is shown in Fig. 25-5F (lifting heel) and Fig. 25-5B (moving leg).

Next turn **body** 90° to your left, pivot on **(L) toes** and pull (L) hip in. Rotate both wrists so both **palms** face outward (Fig. 25-6).

Finally, abduct **(R) shoulder** and pull (R) arm back while you simultaneously extend **(L) elbow.** This latter move will let (L) forearm hit outward and downward with the edge of (L) palm facing downward. Synchronise the movements of your arms with the extension of the **(L) knee** which will permit you to kick outward. This is done only with the **(L) shin** (Fig. 25-7). Remember that all movements should be executed gently, without employing either haste or force.

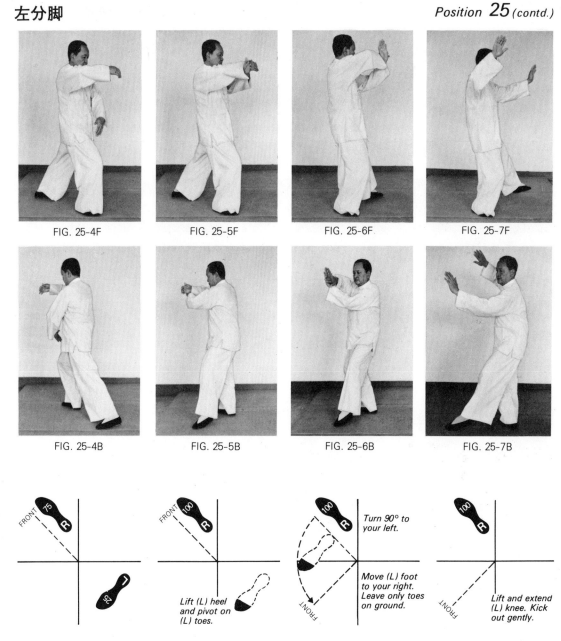

FIG. 25-4F   FIG. 25-5F   FIG. 25-6F   FIG. 25-7F

FIG. 25-4B   FIG. 25-5B   FIG. 25-6B   FIG. 25-7B

Lift (L) heel and pivot on (L) toes.

Turn 90° to your left. Move (L) foot to your right. Leave only toes on ground.

Lift and extend (L) knee. Kick out gently.

Shift entire weight to (R) foot.

转身蹬脚

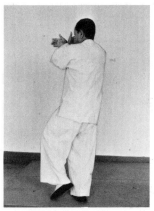

FIG. 26-1F

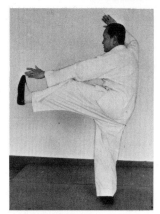

FIG. 26-2F

FIG. 26-3F

Zhǔan shēn dēng jiǎo
Turn and strike with heel

Flex **(L) knee** and pull in (L) shin. This should be done while standing on the **(R) foot.** At the same time pull in both forearms by flexing **elbows.** Then adduct **shoulders** so upper arms sink to your sides. At this point, extend **(R) elbow** so (R) forearm will fall downward and entire (R) arm will hang by your side. Simultaneously, rotate **(L) shoulder** to pull (L) forearm across your body (Fig. 26–1).

Keeping (L) foot suspended in the air, pivot on **(R) heel** and turn **body** and **(R) foot** 135° to your right. The direction **(R) foot** is now pointing should be perpendicular to the direction you are facing. Next abduct both **shoulders** to raise upper arms, then flex **elbows.** This will raise both forearms in front of you. Cross **wrists** with **(R) wrist** on the outside of (L) wrist (Fig. 26–2).

Now abduct **(L) hip** and lift (L) leg till it is parallel to the floor. When you are in this position extend **(L) knee** fully and flex **(L) ankle** so (L) toes point upward. At the same time, rotate both **wrists** so both open palms now face outward. Then extend **(L) elbow** to allow **fingers** to lightly touch raised (L) toes. Simultaneously, stretch **(R) shoulder,** pull it back and, when it is fully abducted, extend **(R) elbow** to lift (R) forearm to an upright position (Fig. 26–3).

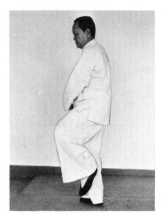

FIG. 26-1B

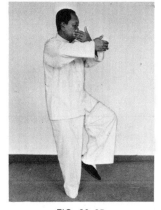

FIG. 26-2B

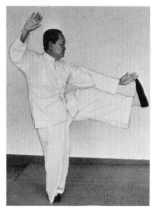

FIG. 26-3B

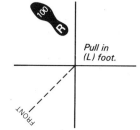

100 R

*Pull in
(L) foot.*

FRONT

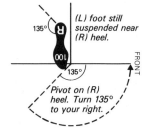

135° R

135°

100

FRONT

*(L) foot still
suspended near
(R) heel.*

*Pivot on (R)
heel. Turn 135°
to your right.*

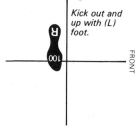

R

100

FRONT

*Kick out and
up with (L)
foot.*

Keep weight on (R) foot.

Zuǒ lǒu xī aǒ bù

Brush left knee and pivot step

When you have completed your kick flex **(L) knee** and pull in (L) shin. Keeping it suspended near the (R) foot, **turn 45°** to your right. At the same time pull (R) arm back in this manner: adduct **(R) shoulder** to bring upper arm back toward your body, rotate **(R) wrist** to turn (R) palm so it faces you, and finally flex **(R) elbow** to bring (R) forearm toward you, with forearm parallel to the ground. Note that **(R) elbow** is still raised and in line with (R) shoulder. Simultaneously, rotate **(L) wrist** to turn **(L) palm** downward, then flex **(L) elbow** to bring (L) forearm toward you, with forearm parallel to the ground (Fig. 27–1).

Step forward and place **(L) foot** down, perpendicular to (R) foot. Keep most of your weight on the back (R) foot. At the same time, adduct **(L) shoulder** and extend **(L) elbow** to bring (L) arm down with **(L) palm** above (R) knee. Keep (R) hand still (Fig. 27–2).

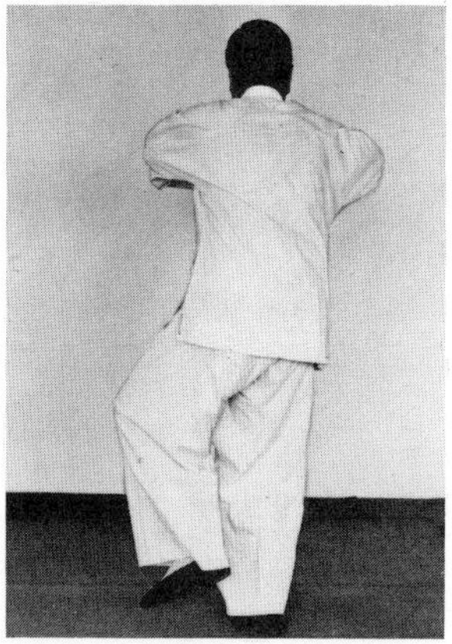

FIG. 27-1F

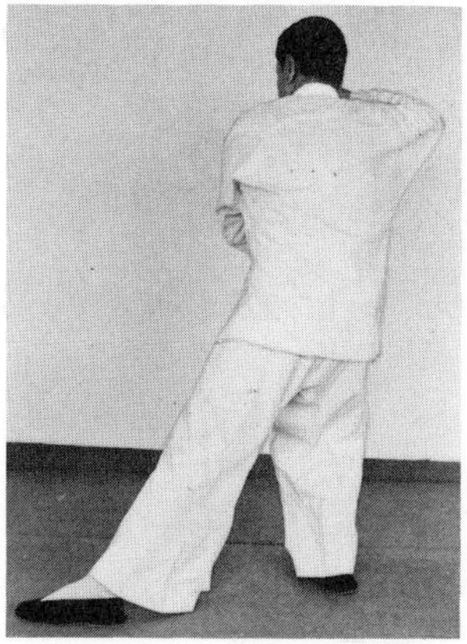

FIG. 27-2F

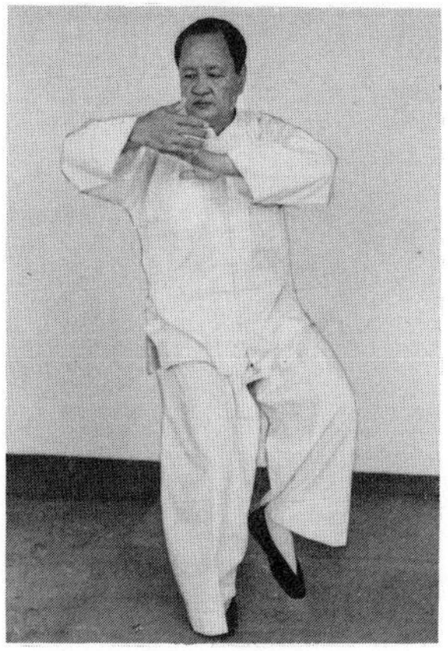

FIG. 27-1B

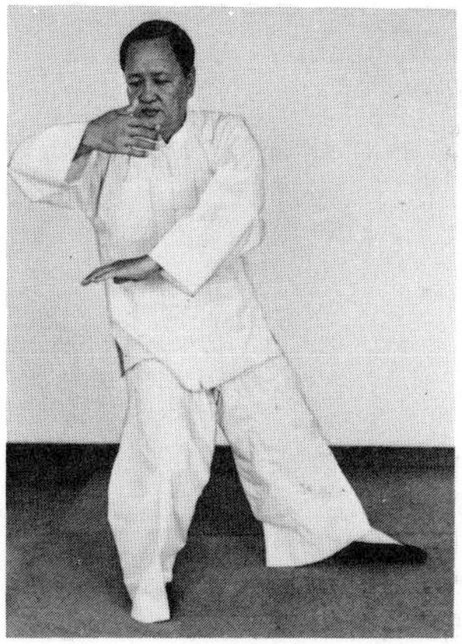

FIG. 27-2B

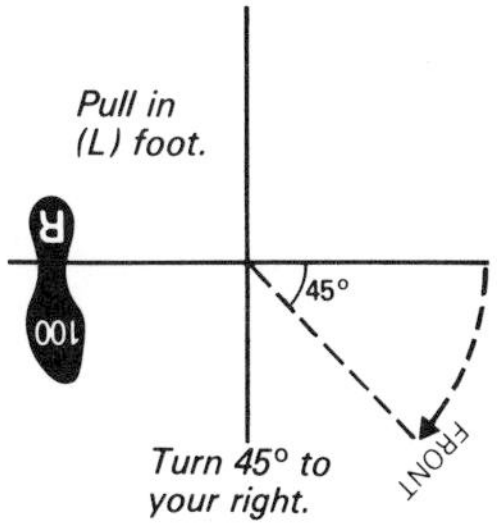

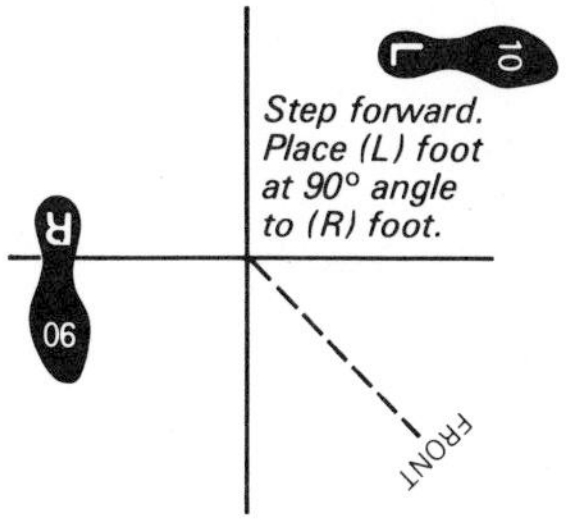

Pull in (L) foot.

Turn 45° to your right.

Step forward. Place (L) foot at 90° angle to (R) foot.

Gradually transfer weight to front (L) foot.

左搂膝拗步

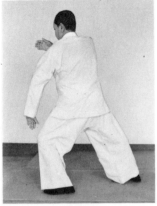

FIG. 27-3F

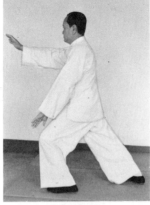

FIG. 27-4F

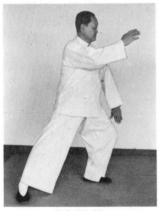

FIG. 27-3B

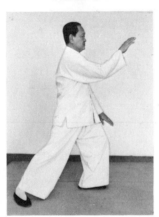

FIG. 27-4B

Zuǒ lǒu xī aǒ bù

Brush left knee and pivot step

Now move (R) arm and simultaneously straighten (R) leg to transfer weight gradually onto front (L) foot. Adduct **(R) shoulder** to bring (R) elbow down till it points to the ground and then abduct **(R) shoulder** to carry arm forward. Notice how Chia keeps (R) elbow away from his body as he executes this hand movement. Use the forward movement of **(R) elbow** to stretch (R) shoulder. Synchronise this with the extension of **(L) elbow** that will permit (L) forearm to sweep downward and forward across your body (Fig. 27-3).

Finally **turn** 45° to your left. Straighten (R) leg and transfer weight onto front **(L) foot.** Turn **(R) foot** 45° to your left and keep it flat on the ground. As you complete the turn, pull in **(L) hip** and pull up **coccyx** so body will be straight and the thrust is directed down to your legs. As (R) arm sweeps forward, rotate **(R) wrist** to turn palm so it faces forward. Keep all tension out of (R) forearm and ensure that (R) elbow is below and not at the same level as your wrist. Remember to extend **fingers** to keep them straight and apart from each other. Keep **(L) elbow** extended so (L) arm will now lie by (L) knee (Fig. 27-4).

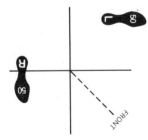

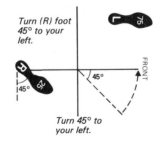

Turn (R) foot
45° to your
left.

Turn 45° to
your left.

Shift weight to front (L) foot.

Yòu lǒu xī aǒ bù
Brush right knee and pivot step

This is essentially a repetition of the last move except that now you use (L) and not (R) hand to hit out.

Initially, relax **(R) hip** and straighten (L) leg in order to move back and shift most of your weight onto back **(R) foot.** Keep **(L) foot** flat on the ground and both arms still (Fig. 28–1).

Now, keeping your weight on back **(R) foot,** pivot on **(L) heel** and turn **(L)** foot 90° to your left. Simultaneously, turn **body** 45° to your left. Extend **(L) shoulder** and, keeping (L) elbow extended, lift entire (L) arm away from your body. Do not move (L) arm backward but lift it sideways (laterally) so it will still be in line with your shoulder. At the same time, flex **(R) elbow** to bring (R) forearm toward you with **(R) palm** facing downward (Fig. 28–2).

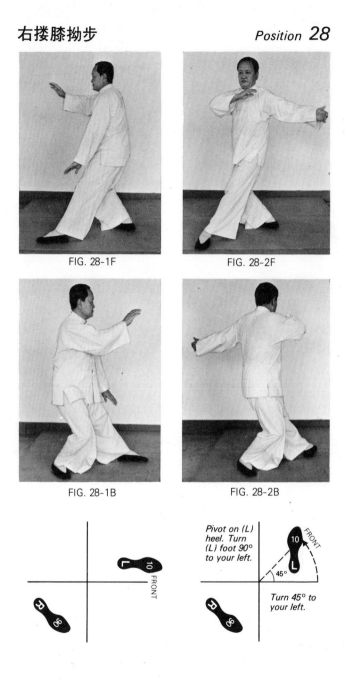

FIG. 28-1F

FIG. 28-2F

FIG. 28-1B

FIG. 28-2B

Pivot on (L) heel. Turn (L) foot 90° to your left.

45°

FRONT

Turn 45° to your left.

FRONT

Move back. Shift weight to back (R) foot.

右搂膝拗步

Yòu lǒu xī aǒ bù
Brush right knee and pivot step

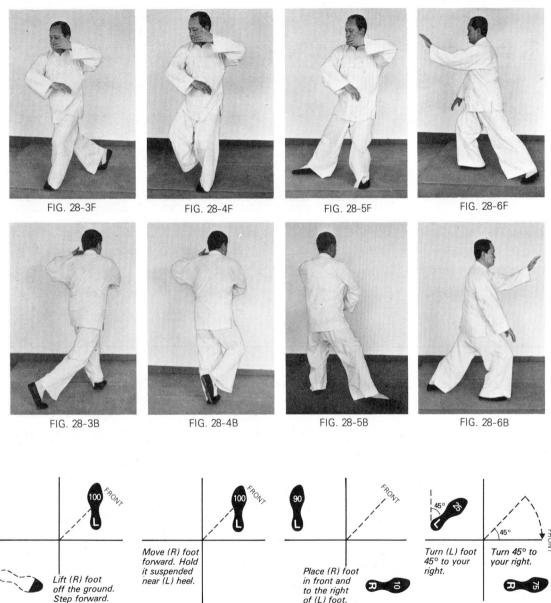

FIG. 28-3F

FIG. 28-4F

FIG. 28-5F

FIG. 28-6F

FIG. 28-3B

FIG. 28-4B

FIG. 28-5B

FIG. 28-6B

Lift (R) foot off the ground. Step forward.

Move (R) foot forward. Hold it suspended near (L) heel.

Place (R) foot in front and to the right of (L) foot.

Turn (L) foot 45° to your right.

Turn 45° to your right.

Shift weight to front (R) foot.

Now move forward, lifting **(R) heel** off the ground and transferring entire weight to **(L) foot.** Simultaneously, flex **(L) elbow** to bring (L) forearm toward you with (L) palm facing your ear (Fig. 28-3). Next lift **(R) foot** off the ground. Move it forward and hold it suspended near (L) heel. All your weight should still be on the (L) foot (Fig. 28-4).

Place your **(R) foot** in front and about a shoulder width to the right of your (L) foot. Set (R) foot down, heel first, and note that it should now be perpendicular to the (L) foot. Do not move either arm at this point (Fig. 28-5).

Finally **turn** 45° to your right, straighten (L) leg and shift your weight onto front **(R) foot.** The **(L) foot** should also turn 45° to your right, to form an angle of 45° with the (R) foot. Simultaneously, extend **(R) elbow** to permit (R) forearm to fall downward till it lies by your (R) knee. Adduct, then abduct **(L) shoulder** to bring (L) arm in front of you. Keep **(L) elbow** extended and rotate **(L) wrist** to turn (L) palm forward. Pull in **(R) hip** so that your body faces the front squarely. Your (L) palm should now be in front of the centre of your chest. The movements of both arms should be well coordinated with the shifting of your weight so they take place just as you move forward (Fig. 28-6).

进步栽捶

Jìn bù zāi chuí

Step forward and strike with fist

This begins with relaxing the **(L) hip** and moving back to put most of your weight onto back **(L) foot.** Do not move either arm (Fig. 29–1).

Now, still keeping weight on the **(L) foot** and, with both arms still, pivot on (R) heel to turn **(R) foot** 90° to your right (Fig. 29–2).

Next move forward, lift **(L) heel** off the ground and **turn** 45° to bring entire weight onto front **(R) foot.** Do not move either arm (Fig. 29–3). Notice that throughout the initial three parts of this move you have not moved either arm in relation to your body.

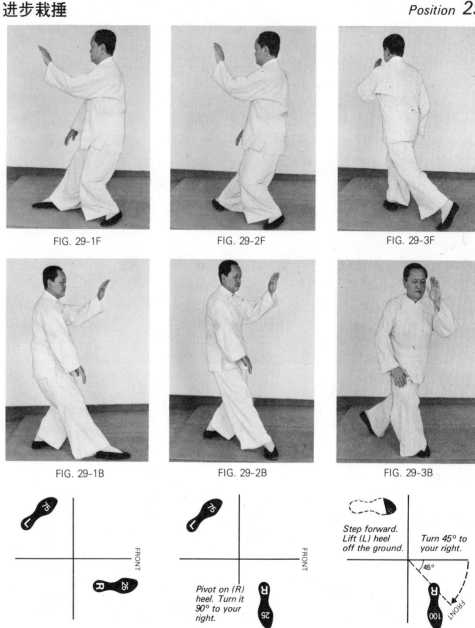

FIG. 29-1F

FIG. 29-2F

FIG. 29-3F

FIG. 29-1B

FIG. 29-2B

FIG. 29-3B

FRONT

Pivot on (R) heel. Turn it 90° to your right.

FRONT

Step forward. Lift (L) heel off the ground.

Turn 45° to your right.

45°

FRONT

Settle back. Then move forward and transfer weight to front (R) foot.

进步栽捶

Jìn bù zāi chuí

Step forward and strike with fist

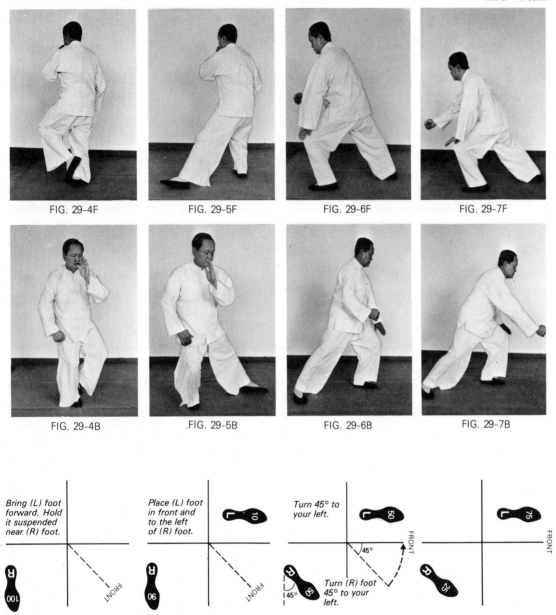

FIG. 29-4F　　FIG. 29-5F　　FIG. 29-6F　　FIG. 29-7F

FIG. 29-4B　　FIG. 29-5B　　FIG. 29-6B　　FIG. 29-7B

Bring (L) foot forward. Hold it suspended near (R) foot.

Place (L) foot in front and to the left of (R) foot.

Turn 45° to your left.

Turn (R) foot 45° to your left.

Step out. Transfer weight to front (L) foot.

The next four parts of this move involve you stepping forward and executing a low punch. Initially, lift the **(L) foot** off the ground, bring it forward and hold it suspended near the (R) foot. At the same time clench **(R) hand** to form a fist while keeping (L) arm and hand still (Fig. 29–4).

Step out and place **(L) foot** in front of the (R) foot. (L) foot should point forward and be at right angles to (R) foot. Concentrate weight on back **(R) foot.** Look downward and forward (Fig. 29–5).

Next, straighten **(R) leg** and **turn** 45° to your left to bring your weight onto the **(L) foot.** Rotate **(L) shoulder** and then extend **(L) elbow** to permit (L) forearm to sweep across your body. The (L) hand will lie beside the (L) knee with **(L) palm** facing away from you. Keep **eyes** focused on an imaginary object on the ground in front.

Finally, pull in **(L) hip** completely and turn **(R) foot** 45° to your left. This turn will bring the (L) arm more to the left and rotate the (L) palm so that it faces downward (Fig. 29–6). At the same time bend **spine** slightly and extend **(R) elbow** to punch downward and forward with clenched (R) fist. Keep eyes focused on (R) fist. Do not lean forward too much and ensure that (L) knee is in line with (L) toes (Fig. 29–7). If you had executed this move correctly you would have felt an increased load on (L) thigh muscles and tension on (L) knee.

Shàng bù, lǎn què wěi

Step forward, grasp sparrow's tail

上步揽雀尾

This move is essentially similar to that described for Position 4 (pages 24–27).

Straighten **(L) leg** and **spine** to move back and assume an upright stance. At the same time, bring most of your weight back onto **(R) foot**. Simultaneously, unclench **(R) fist** and then adduct **(R) shoulder** to bring (R) arm back to your side with open (R) palm facing downward. Raise **(L) arm** to shoulder level, then flex **(L) elbow** to pull **(L) forearm** toward you. Your **(L) palm** should face you (Fig. 30–1).

Then, keeping arms still and weight on back **(R) foot**, pivot on **(L) heel** and turn (L) foot 90° to your left. Now lift **(R) heel** off the ground, move forward and **turn** 45° to your left, transferring your weight onto front (L) foot. At the same time adduct **(L) shoulder** to pull (L) arm toward you with (L) elbow pointing downward. Keep **(L) elbow** flexed so (L) palm now faces forward. Extend **(L) wrist** slightly so hand and forearm are in a straight line. Simultaneously rotate **(R) wrist** and flex **(R) elbow** slightly. Your (R) forearm will then be pulled toward your body with (R) palm facing you (Fig. 30–2).

Finally move forward. Lift **(R) foot** forward and hold it suspended near the (L) foot (Fig. 30–3).

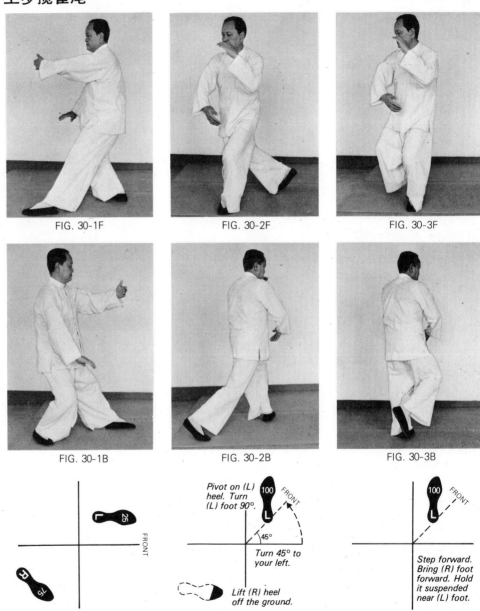

FIG. 30-1F   FIG. 30-2F   FIG. 30-3F

FIG. 30-1B   FIG. 30-2B   FIG. 30-3B

Pivot on (L) heel. Turn (L) foot 90°.

Turn 45° to your left.

Lift (R) heel off the ground.

Step forward. Bring (R) foot forward. Hold it suspended near (L) foot.

Settle back. Then step forward and transfer weight to front (L) foot.

上步揽雀尾（棚手）

Shàng bù, lǎn què wěi (péng shǒu)

Step forward, grasp sparrow's tail, ward off

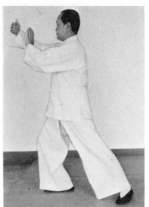

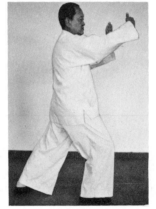

FIG. 30-4F   FIG. 30-5F   FIG. 30-6F

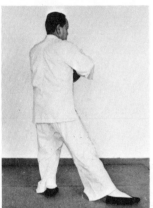
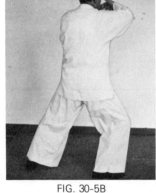

FIG. 30-4B   FIG. 30-5B   FIG. 30-6B

This series of moves is essentially similar to those for Position 4, *lǎn què wěi (péng shǒu),* described earlier on page 24.

Initially, bring **(R) foot** forward and place it in front of and perpendicular to (L) foot. Place (R) foot as far forward as you can while maintaining the bulk of your weight on back **(L) foot.** Keep both arms still at this point (Fig. 30–4).

Now straighten (L) leg to move forward and gradually transfer weight onto (R) foot. At the same time abduct **(R) shoulder** to raise (R) arm. Then, holding (R) arm still, rotate **(R) shoulder** to bring (R) upper arm to a vertical position, i.e., turn (R) elbow through 90° so it points downward. Keep **(R) elbow** flexed and (R) palm at eye level. Keep (L) arm still (Fig. 30–5).

Continue transferring weight onto front (R) foot and **turn** 45° to your right. As you do this allow **(L) foot** to follow the move and turn through 45° to your right at the same time. Keep hands still in front of you with both palms facing each other. Pull in your **pelvis** and **(R) hip** and maintain a straight posture (Fig. 30–6).

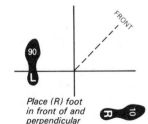

Place (R) foot in front of and perpendicular to (L) foot.

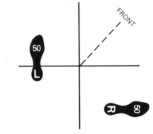

Turn 45° to your right.

Move (L) foot 45° to your right.

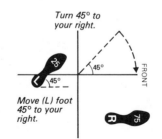

Shift weight to front (R) foot.

Shàng bù, lǎn què wěi (lí shǒu)

Step forward, grasp sparrow's tail, roll back

This is similar to the part of Position 4, *lǎn què wěi*, that was described in some detail on page 25. On this page we will highlight the more important aspects of the move.

There are two distinct parts to *lí shǒu*. The first basically involves **moving back,** transferring weight to the back (L) foot. The important thing to look out for in carrying out this move, is to ensure that you move as far back as you can while maintaining a straight posture (Fig. 30–7). This should be accomplished before initiating the second part of this move — **turning** 45° to your left (Fig. 30–8). Do not turn before you have moved back completely; if you do your weight would fall midway between your legs and you can then be made to lose your balance rather easily.

The other point to note is that the sole of the front (R) foot should remain flat on the ground as you shift weight back. Remember also to pull in your (R) hip so that the hips are in line with the shoulders. This would increase the tension on your legs and create the tendency for you to lift your (R) toes off the ground. Guard against this.

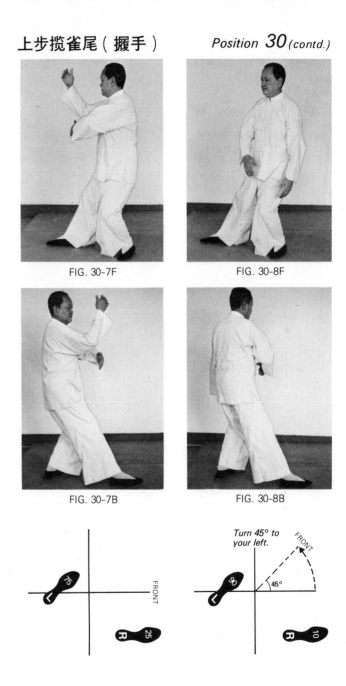

FIG. 30-7F

FIG. 30-8F

FIG. 30-7B

FIG. 30-8B

Turn 45° to your left.

Shift weight to back (L) foot.

上步揽雀尾（挤手）

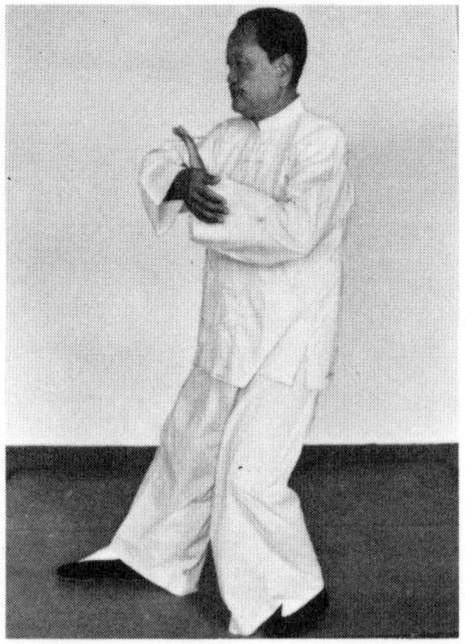

FIG. 30-9F

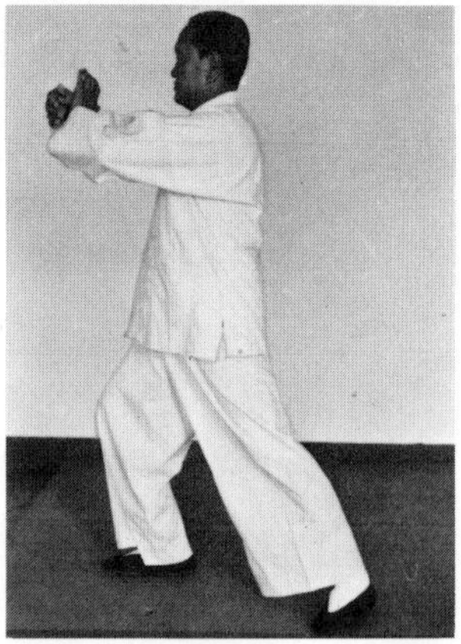

FIG. 30-10F

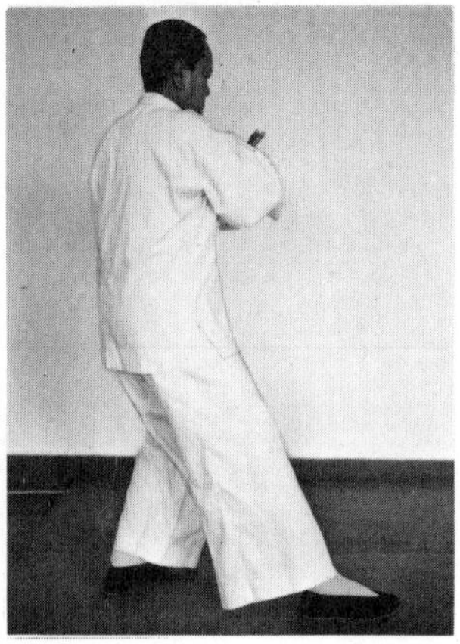

FIG. 30-9B

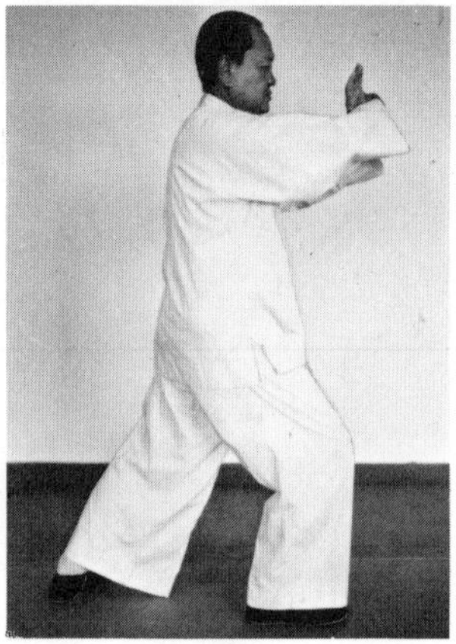

FIG. 30-10B

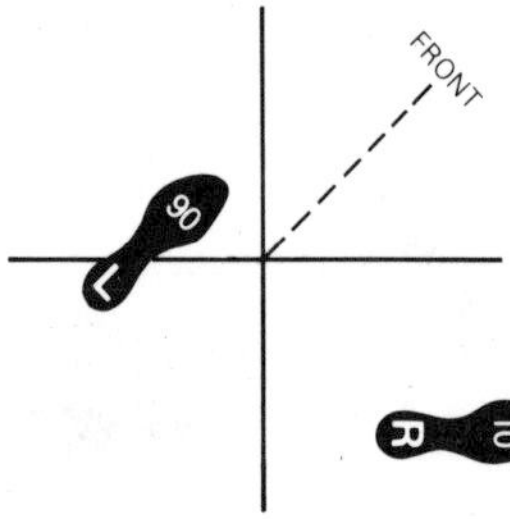

FRONT

90
L

R
10

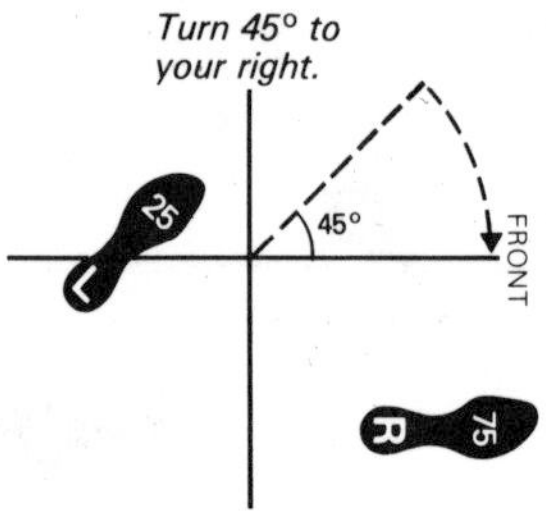

Turn 45° to
your right.

25
L

45°

FRONT

R
75

Move forward. Transfer weight to front (R) foot.

Shàng bù, lǎn què wěi (jǐ shǒu)

Step forward, grasp sparrow's tail, press

This is similar to *jǐ shǒu* of *lǎn què wěi*, illustrated and described on page 26.

This move can also be described in two parts. The first involves pressing **(L) palm** against inner part of **(R) wrist** (while maintaining weight on back **(L) foot**) and the second involves moving forward, transferring weight onto front **(R) foot** and turning **body** 45° to your right.

Note that the pressing of (L) palm against (R) wrist takes place **while** you are still resting on the back (L) foot. Do not carry out this manoeuvre while moving forward (Fig. 30–9).

Another point to remember is that the thrust forward is produced by straightening the (L) leg. The force should not come from either shoulders or arms which should be relaxed and free from tension (Fig. 30–10). Thus the direction of the thrust would be forward and upward. If the thrust had originated from either shoulders or elbows, its direction would be either straight forward or forward and downward.

Finally, remember to turn your **waist** 45° to your right as you complete the move. This would also provide an additional impetus to your thrust while your hands remain passive and relaxed.

Shàng bù, lǎn què wěi (àn shǒu)

Step forward, grasp sparrow's tail, push down

This is similar to *àn shǒu* of *lǎn què wěi*, described on page 27. The first part of this move essentially involves moving back and resting on the back **(L) leg.** In your move back, try to maintain as straight a posture as possible. Avoid moving either back or head before or after the rest of the body. It is important to move the entire body back as one complete unit (Fig. 30–11).

The other aspect that you would have to pay particular attention to in this move is the movement of arms. Initially, adduct both **shoulders,** so elbows sink downward toward the floor.

Avoid keeping elbows either behind your body or splayed out in front of you as you thrust forward (Fig. 30–12). The objective of this manoeuvre is to utilise the power of your (L) leg to generate the force for your forward thrust. It is, therefore, important to relax arms completely and not to push from your arms as you move forward. You can only effectively utilise power from your legs and bring it up to your palms when this is achieved. Keeping arms relaxed is also important in combat as it will permit you to respond very quickly to any counter-attack.

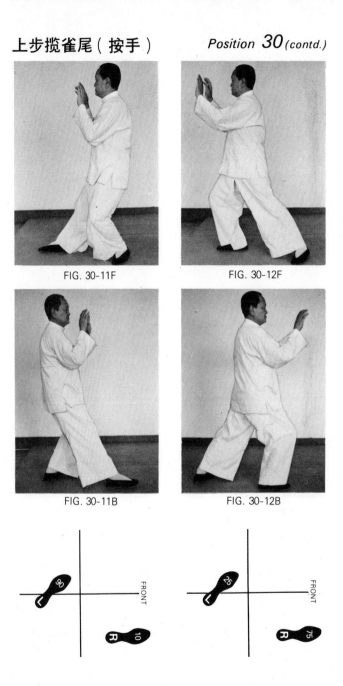

FIG. 30-11F

FIG. 30-12F

FIG. 30-11B

FIG. 30-12B

Move back onto back (L) foot, then forward onto front (R) foot.

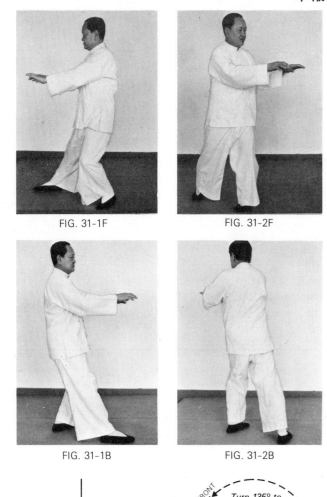

FIG. 31-1F　　　　　　　　FIG. 31-2F

FIG. 31-1B　　　　　　　　FIG. 31-2B

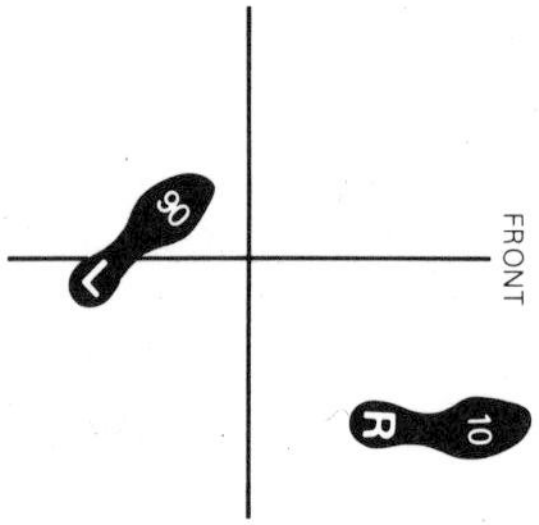

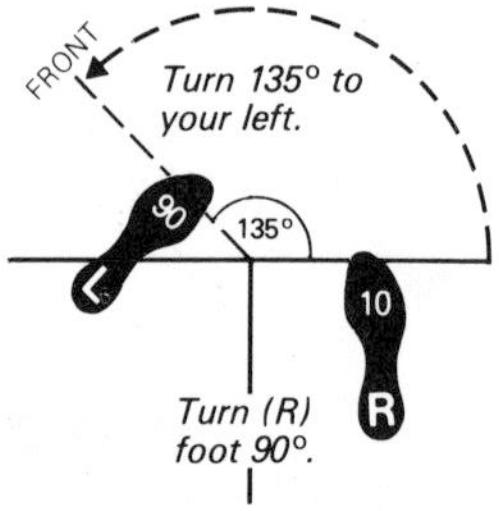

Turn 135° to your left.

135°

Turn (R) foot 90°.

Transfer weight to back (L) foot.

Dān biān
Single whip

The moves which initiate the concluding position for Chapter Three were described on page 28. They illustrate the link movements that enable you to move from the last position to this one.

Fig. 31–1 illustrates that you would relax the **(L) hip** to move backward and settle on back **(L) foot**.

Fig. 31–2 illustrates the 135° **turn** to your left. Two features particularly must be remembered in executing this turn. First it should be carried out at your **waist.** Do not execute the turn with only forearms, with waist kept still.

The next thing to remember is **not** to turn your (R) foot simultaneously with your waist. Turn body as much as you can first. Only when you have some difficulty do you allow your **(R) foot** to start turning 90° to your left. The turning of the (R) foot should start approximately when you have turned your body through about 45° so that both body and foot would complete their turn at the same time (you turn your body through 135° and your foot through only 90°). Keep your weight on **(L) foot** while making this turn.

单鞭

Dān biān

Single whip

The three moves illustrated here are a repetition of moves which you have done earlier. Detailed descriptions of these moves have been presented on page 29.

The first of the three moves involves shifting weight from (L) to **(R) foot** and pulling in both **forearms** so palms face each other (Fig. 31–3). The next two moves involve **turning** 135° to your right (Fig. 31–4) and completely extending **(R) elbow** (Fig. 31–5). Throughout the turn remember to keep your weight on one leg — this time on your (R) foot.

As in the initial part of this move, it is important to remember that the turn is carried out at your **waist** with both arms lying passively in front of you. Your arms, however, should not be held too close to your body but some distance away. Keep the **(R) shoulder** abducted in order to hold (R) upper arm away from your body.

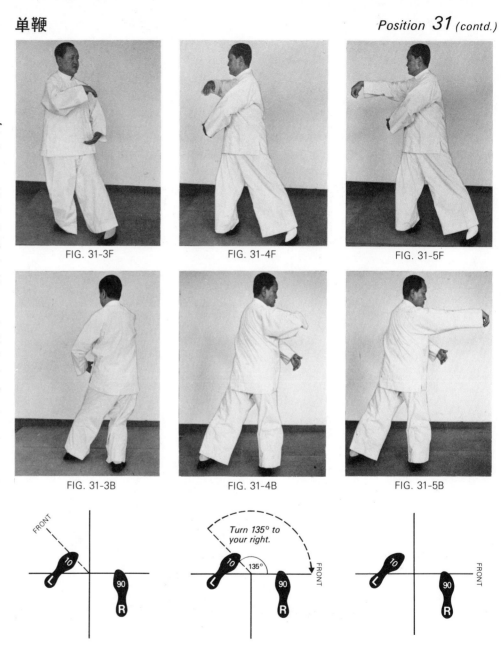

FIG. 31-3F   FIG. 31-4F   FIG. 31-5F

FIG. 31-3B   FIG. 31-4B   FIG. 31-5B

Turn 135° to your right.

Move back. Transfer weight to (R) foot.

单鞭

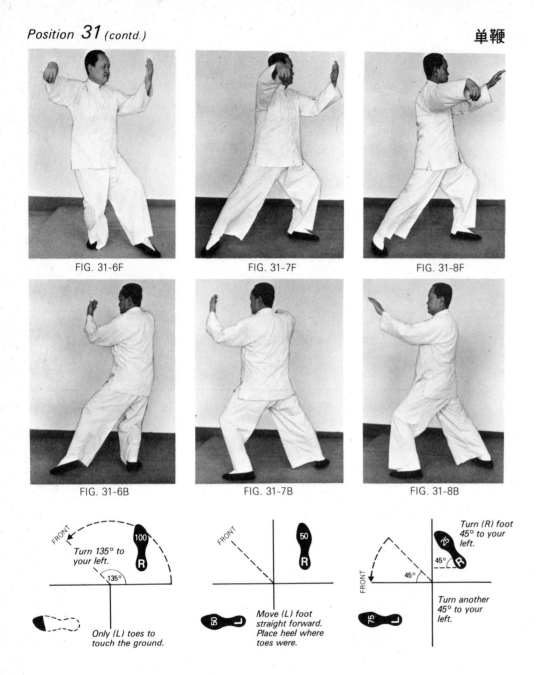

FIG. 31-6F   FIG. 31-7F   FIG. 31-8F

FIG. 31-6B   FIG. 31-7B   FIG. 31-8B

Turn 135° to your left.

Only (L) toes to touch the ground.

Move (L) foot straight forward. Place heel where toes were.

Turn (R) foot 45° to your left.

Turn another 45° to your left.

Move forward. Transfer weight to (L) foot.

Dān biān
Single whip

A detailed description of the completion of *dān biān* is given on page 30.

A detailed description of the completion of *dān biān* is given on page 30.

A common error in positioning (Figs. 31–1 to 31–7) is to turn your head either before or after turning your body. In order to avoid this, focus your vision on the (L) palm throughout: this will help you coordinate the movement of your head with your body. While executing the turn, keep your weight focused on back (R) foot. Before you start shifting your weight forward onto the (L) foot, ensure that it is placed down flat on the ground first. Do not move forward with your (L) foot still in the air. In combat, this would make it very easy for an opponent to upset your balance.

The most difficult part to master in *dān biān* is the last move. The main difficulty lies in pulling in your pelvis to keep your torso straight. It is not possible to achieve this correct posture in a short space of time and you need to correct yourself gradually as you continue practising and developing greater power in your legs. You should have noticed that all the turns executed (for this and for other moves) of either body or feet are always through an angle of 45° or multiples of 45° – 90°, 135°, 180°.

This concludes the third part of the exercise. You might note that the first three chapters of the taiji exercise end with *dān biān*.

Chapter Four

This chapter consists of thirteen moves of which six are new and seven are moves covered earlier. Some of the most difficult moves are, quite appropriately, only introduced in this chapter.

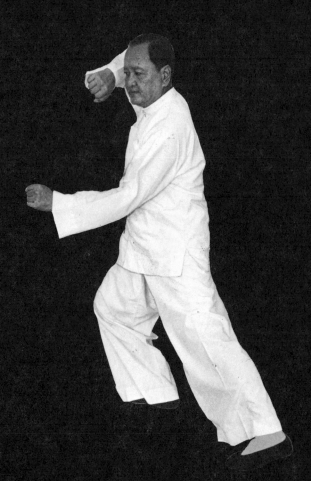

玉女穿梭

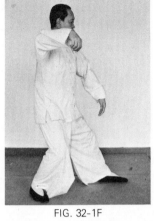

FIG. 32-1F

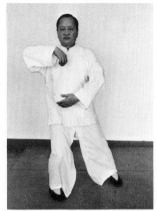

FIG. 32-2F

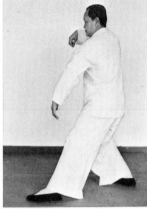

FIG. 32-1B

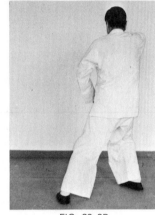

FIG. 32-2B

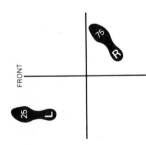

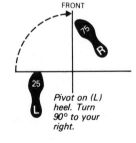

Pivot on (L) heel. Turn 90° to your right.

Settle back. Keep weight on (R) foot.

Yù nǚ chuān suō

Fair lady works at shuttles

This is a complex move that is illustrated in a series of 27 pictures, presented over pages 96–104. Basically, it shows how you can turn to face four different directions, all at an angle of 180° to each other. For instance, if you had begun facing the side of a room, then you will turn to face all four corners of that room during this move.

Initially settle back to transfer weight onto back **(R) foot.** At the same time adduct **(L) shoulder** and, keeping **(L) elbow** extended, pull (L) arm toward your body. Keep (R) hand flexed and still at this stage (Fig. 32–1).

Next pivot on **(L) heel** and simultaneously turn both (L) foot and **body** 90° to your right. At the same time flex both **elbows.** This will bring (R) forearm toward your body and, as **(R) shoulder** is still abducted, the upper (R) arm is held away from your body. Your (R) forearm will be in line with both upper arm and shoulder with (R) palm facing downward. Flexion of **(L) elbow** will pull (L) forearm toward your body with (L) palm facing upward (Fig. 32–2).

Yù nǚ chuān suō

Fair lady works at shuttles

The next six pictures on pages 97–98 illustrate the moves involved which permit you to turn 135° to your right.

First, relax **(L) hip,** straighten (R) leg to move back and focus weight on back **(L) foot.** Do not move either arm (Fig. 32–3).

Now, keeping entire weight on the **(L) foot,** lift **(R) foot** off the ground and move it toward your right. Place it in front of and perpendicular to the (L) heel. Keep most of your weight on the **(L) foot.** At the same time turn **body** 45° to your right and adduct **(R) shoulder** to pull (R) upper arm toward you with (R) elbow pointing downward. Keep **(R) elbow** flexed so (R) forearm is now in an upright position. Extend **(R) wrist** to raise (R) palm and keep fingers straight (Fig. 32–4).

Next lift **(L) heel** off the ground and transfer weight onto front **(R) foot.** At the same time **turn** another 45° to your right so you will now face the direction your (R) foot is pointing (Fig. 32–5).

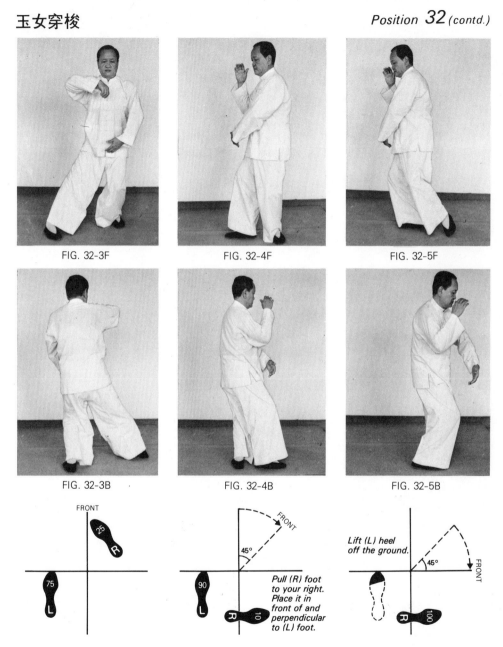

FIG. 32-3F   FIG. 32-4F   FIG. 32-5F

FIG. 32-3B   FIG. 32-4B   FIG. 32-5B

Pull (R) foot to your right. Place it in front of and perpendicular to (L) foot.

Lift (L) heel off the ground.

Initially settle back on (L) foot. Then transfer weight to (R) foot.

玉女穿梭

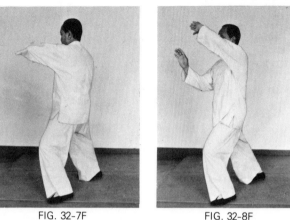
FIG. 32-7F

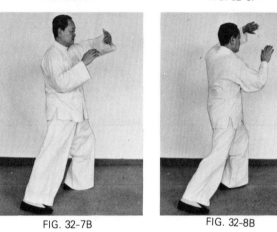
FIG. 32-6F

FIG. 32-8F

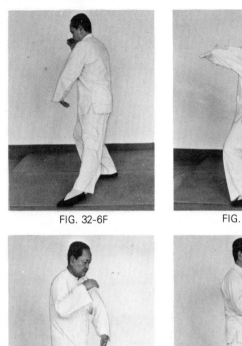
FIG. 32-6B

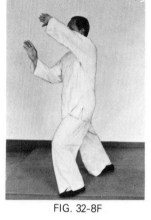
FIG. 32-7B

FIG. 32-8B

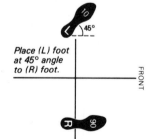

10
L
45°

*Place (L) foot
at 45° angle
to (R) foot.*

FRONT

R
90

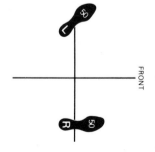

50
L

FRONT

R
50

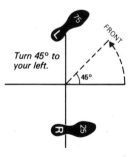

75
L

*Turn 45° to
your left.*

FRONT

45°

R
25

Yù nǚ chuān suō

Fair lady works at shuttles

Now move **(L) leg** to your left and place it so (L) heel is in line with and points 45° toward the left of the (R) foot. Keep weight on **(R) foot** and arms still at this stage (Fig. 32–6).

Next straighten back **(R) foot** and begin the transfer of weight to front **(L) foot.** As you accomplish this, abduct **(L) shoulder** and keep **(L) elbow** flexed to lift (L) arm. At this point, (L) forearm is perpendicular to (L) upper arm and **(L) palm** faces you (Fig. 32–7).

Finally **turn** 45° to your left, and at the same time straighten back **(R) leg** to shift more weight onto front (L) foot. Abduct **(R) shoulder** to thrust (R) arm forward in front of you, keeping **(R) elbow** flexed so (R) forearm is upright with elbow below the hand and palm facing forward. As you carry out this manoeuvre, continue to adduct **(L) elbow** further to raise (L) forearm till it is held away from your body at slightly higher than eye level. At this point rotate **(L) wrist** so (L) palm now faces forward. You would, by now, be facing one corner, at an angle of 135° to the right from where you were initially facing at the beginning of the move (Figs. 32–1 and 32–8).

Shift weight to front (L) foot.

Yù nǚ chuān suō

Fair lady works at shuttles

The next six pictures on pages 99–100 show how you would be able to execute a move that is the mirror image of the previous one. You will turn through 270° to face a different corner from the last (Fig. 32-8).

The first three figures (Figs. 32-9 to 32-11) illustrate how you would execute part of the turn. Initially, relax **(R) hip** and move back to bring most of your weight onto the **(R) foot.** At the same time adduct **(L) shoulder** to draw (L) upper arm inward with (L) elbow pointing downward. Keep **(L) elbow** flexed so (L) forearm is upright with open **(L) palm** facing your right. Simultaneously, adduct **(R) shoulder,** pull in (R) upper arm till (R) elbow is by your side. Then abduct **(R) shoulder** to raise upper arm laterally (sideways) and to bring (R) hand below (L) elbow. At this point, **(R) forearm** is parallel to the ground and **(R) palm** faces downward (Fig. 32-9).

Next turn both **body** and **(L) foot** 90° to your right, keeping weight on **(R) foot** and arms still (Fig. 32-10).

Finally, straighten **(R) leg** to put entire weight on **(L) foot.** Lift **(R) heel** off the ground and, pivoting on **(R) toes,** turn another 45° to your right. By now, you would have turned a total of 135° to your right. Keep both arms still (Fig. 32-11).

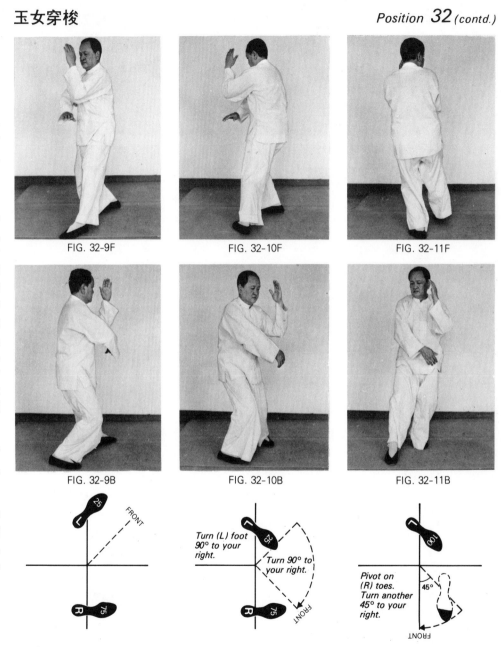

FIG. 32-9F   FIG. 32-10F   FIG. 32-11F

FIG. 32-9B   FIG. 32-10B   FIG. 32-11B

Turn (L) foot 90° to your right.

Turn 90° to your right.

Pivot on (R) toes. Turn another 45° to your right.

First move back onto back (R) foot. Turn 90° and shift back to (L) foot.

玉女穿梭

Yù nǔ chuān suō

Fair lady works at shuttles

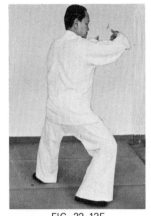

FIG. 32-12F

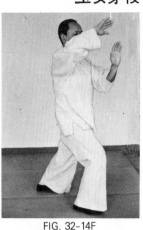

FIG. 32-13F

FIG. 32-14F

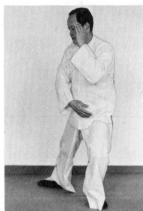

FIG. 32-12B

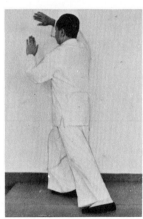

FIG. 32-13B

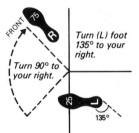

FIG. 32-14B

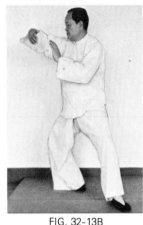

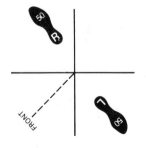

Turn 45° to your right.

Place (R) foot in line with and pointing away from (L) foot.

45°

FRONT

Turn 90° to your right.

FRONT

Turn (L) foot 135° to your right.

FRONT

135°

Shift weight to front (L) foot.

Lift **(R) foot** slightly off the ground and move it to your right, placing it as far as possible at an angle of 180° to the (L) foot. Both feet should, at this stage, point in opposite directions. In order to facilitate the proper positioning of your feet, you have to **turn** another 45° to your right. Keep arms still and weight on **(L) foot** (Fig. 32-12).

While facing the same direction, straighten (L) leg to gradually begin the transfer of weight onto the **(R) foot.** As you move forward, abduct **(R) shoulder** and lift (R) upper arm away from your body. Keep **(R) elbow** flexed so (R) forearm is at right angles to (R) upper arm and both palms now face each other (Fig. 32-13).

Finally **turn** another 90° to your right. This should be coordinated with a 135° turn of the **(L) foot** to your right. Your (R) foot should now be at a 45° angle to the (L) foot. Straighten (L) leg and pull in **(R) hip** to bring weight onto front **(R) foot.** At the same time abduct **(L) shoulder** to thrust (L) arm forward. Keep (R) arm still. At the completion of the turn rotate **(R) wrist** to turn (R) palm forward. Note that at this point the front (R) foot, both palms and your body all face the same direction (Fig. 32-14). This brings you to a position which is the mirror image of Fig. 32-8. In this instance, the (R) foot and (L) arm are in front.

Yù nǚ chuān suō

Fair lady works at shuttles

The next six moves on pages 101–102 show how you could turn 90° to your left.

First move back and rest most of your weight on back **(L) foot**. At the same time adduct **(R) shoulder** and pull (R) upper arm toward you till (R) elbow points downward. Keep **(R) elbow** flexed; this will bring (R) forearm to an upright position with **(R) palm** facing your left. Simultaneously, adduct **(L) shoulder** to bring (L) elbow down to your side. Then move (L) forearm toward you and down to your right till it is parallel to the ground with **(L) palm** below (R) elbow and facing downward (Fig. 32-15).

With weight on **(L) foot,** pivot on **(R) heel** and turn (R) foot 45° to your right. Next straighten (L) leg and move forward, bringing most of your weight to bear on front (R) foot (Fig. 32-16). Rotate **(L) wrist** to face palm inward. Lift **(L) foot** off the ground, bring it forward and hold it suspended near the (R) foot (Fig. 32-17). Throughout both these latter moves do not move either arm.

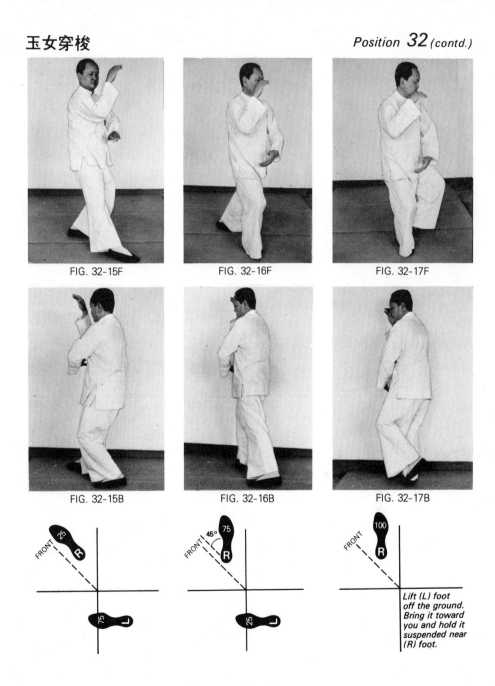

FIG. 32-15F FIG. 32-16F FIG. 32-17F

FIG. 32-15B FIG. 32-16B FIG. 32-17B

Lift (L) foot off the ground. Bring it toward you and hold it suspended near (R) foot.

Initially settle back on back (L) foot then move forward onto front (R) foot.

玉女穿梭

Yù nǚ chuān suō

Fair lady works at shuttles

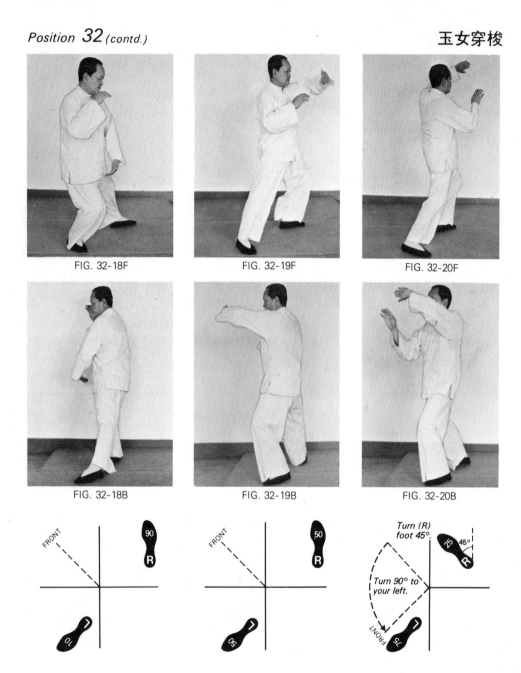

FIG. 32-18F   FIG. 32-19F   FIG. 32-20F

FIG. 32-18B   FIG. 32-19B   FIG. 32-20B

Keeping weight on **(R) foot**, stretch **(L) leg** as far to your left as possible, then place it down (heel first) in front of and at 135° to the (R) foot (Fig. 32–18).

Next straighten back **(R) leg** to gradually transfer the bulk of your weight onto front **(L) foot**. Initially, while facing the same direction, abduct **(L) shoulder** and lift (L) upper arm. Keep **(L) elbow** extended so (L) forearm will be parallel to the ground and at right angles to (L) upper arm (Fig. 32–19).

Finally **turn** 90° to your left so your body faces the direction in which (L) foot points. Coordinate this with the 45° turn to the left by your **(R) foot**. At this point the bulk of your weight should rest on front (L) foot. The turning of your body should also be coordinated with the forward thrust of the (R) hand. This should be carried out by abducting **(R) shoulder** and raising (R) arm forward with **(R) elbow** flexed. Try to keep tension and force out of the (R) forearm. At the completion of your turn, rotate **(L) wrist** so (L) palm now faces forward. Your **(L) palm** should finally be above and behind the **(R) palm** (Fig. 32–20).

Place (L) foot down. Transfer weight onto it.

Yù nǔ chuān suō

Fair lady works at shuttles

This is the last part of a complex move, which brings you to face the fourth corner of the room. It is illustrated on pages 103 and 104 and involves a turn through an angle of 270°.

The pictures on this page illustrate the initial 135° turn. First move back and transfer weight onto back **(R) foot.** As you do this adduct **(L) shoulder** to pull (L) upper arm inward and toward you, till (L) elbow points downward. Your **(L) forearm** will now be upright. At the same time adduct **(R) shoulder** and bring (R) arm toward you until (R) elbow is by your side. Then abduct **(R) shoulder** to raise (R) upper arm sideways and to bring (R) palm down till it is below (L) elbow. Your (R) palm now faces downward (Fig. 32–21). Keep arms still for the next two parts of this move.

With your weight on the **(R) foot,** pivot on **(L) heel** and turn both **body** and **(L) foot** 90° to your right (Fig. 32–22).

Relax **(L) hip,** move backward and rest on **(L) foot.** Next pivot on **(R) heel** and turn both **body** and **(R) foot** 45° to the right. You will now face the direction in which (R) foot points (Fig. 32–23).

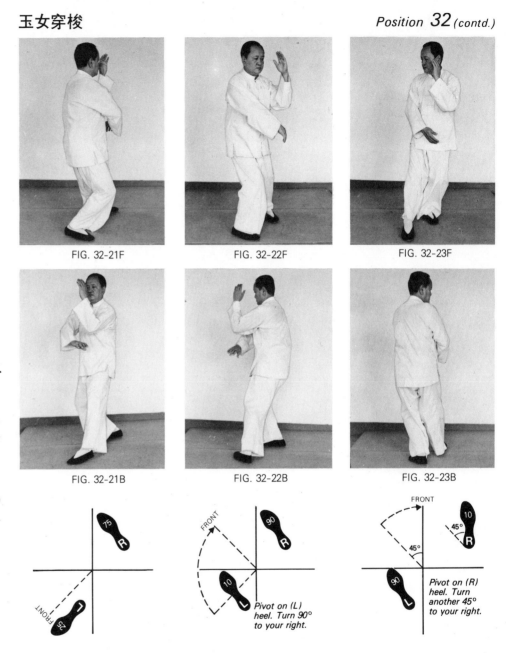

FIG. 32-21F FIG. 32-22F FIG. 32-23F

FIG. 32-21B FIG. 32-22B FIG. 32-23B

Move back onto (R) foot then turn 90° and transfer weight back to (L) foot.

玉女穿梭

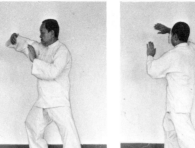

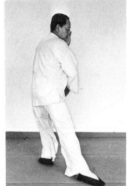

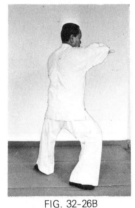

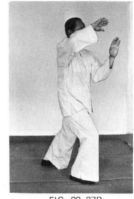

FIG. 32-24F   FIG. 32-25F   FIG. 32-26F   FIG. 32-27F

FIG. 32-24B   FIG. 32-25B   FIG. 32-26B   FIG. 32-27B

Yù nǔ chuān suō

Fair lady works at shuttles

In this last part, first lift **(R) foot** off the ground, flex **(R) knee** and pull (R) shin toward you, holding it suspended near (L) foot. At the same time turn 45° to your right (Fig. 32–24). Keeping weight on (L) foot, stretch **(R) foot** as far right as possible and place it down 180° away from (L) foot. Both heels should be in line. Keep arms still during both these moves (Fig. 32–25).

Next straighten **(L) leg** and raise (R) arm at (R) shoulder (Fig. 32–26). Finally turn **(L) foot** 135° and **body** another 90° to your right. Simultaneously, adduct **(L) shoulder** to thrust (L) arm forward. Co-ordinate this with the rotation of the (R) wrist to turn (R) palm forward. Weight should now be on front (R) foot (Fig. 32–27).

This will turn you through another 270° to end facing the fourth corner of the room. The four parts of this move will, progressively, make you face the four corners if you had begun facing one side of the room (see diagrams below).

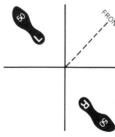

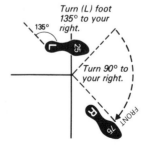

FRONT

Lift (R) foot off the ground. Pull it to (L) foot.

Turn 45° to your right.

Place (R) foot pointing away from (L) foot.

Turn (L) foot 135° to your right.

Turn 90° to your right.

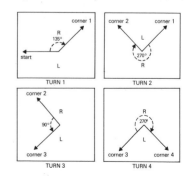

TURN 1   TURN 2

TURN 3   TURN 4

Gradually shift weight to front (R) foot.

Zuǒ péng shǒu

Ward off, left

This is essentially a repetition of Position 3 which was illustrated and described on page 23. The difference lies in the initial link move, where you first have to move back onto your **(L) foot** and bring both arms in.

As you move back, adduct **(R) shoulder** to pull (R) elbow vertically till it points downward. At the same time turn **(L) wrist** so (L) palm faces your right, then adduct **(L) shoulder** to bring (L) forearm toward you. Upon completing this, lift **(L) heel** off the ground and pivot on **(L) toes** to turn (L) foot 90° to your left. This will make the angle between your feet 135°. Keep weight concentrated on the **(R) foot** (Fig. 33–1).

Next **turn** 90° to your left and coordinate this turn with the straightening of the back **(R) leg** to transfer most of your weight onto front **(L) foot.** Simultaneously abduct **(L) shoulder** to lift (L) arm until it is at shoulder level. Keep **(L) elbow** flexed so (L) arm is parallel to the floor with (L) forearm at right angles to (L) upper arm. At the same time extend **(R) elbow** so (R) forearm falls to your side (Fig. 33–2).

Complete the move by **turning** another 45° to your left. This should be synchronised with the turning of the **(R) foot** 90° to your left. Keep arms still in relation to your body. Note that your open **(L) palm** now faces the centre of your chest. Most of your weight should lie on the front **(L) foot** (Fig. 33–3).

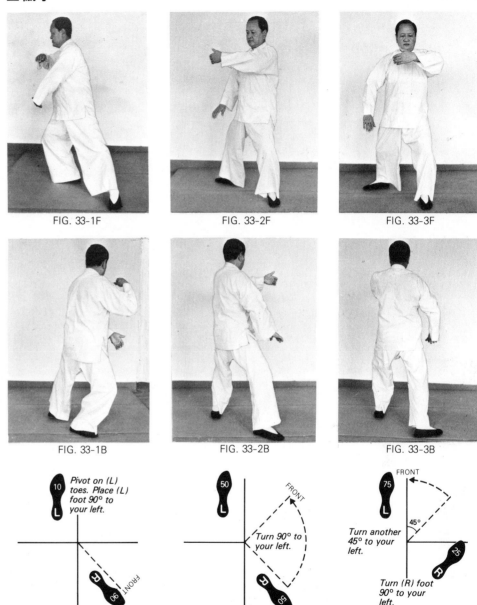

FIG. 33-1F

FIG. 33-2F

FIG. 33-3F

FIG. 33-1B

FIG. 33-2B

FIG. 33-3B

Pivot on (L) toes. Place (L) foot 90° to your left.

Turn 90° to your left.

FRONT

Turn another 45° to your left.

Turn (R) foot 90° to your left.

Transfer weight to (L) foot.

揽雀尾（棚手）

Lǎn què wěi (péng shǒu)

Grasp sparrow's tail, ward off

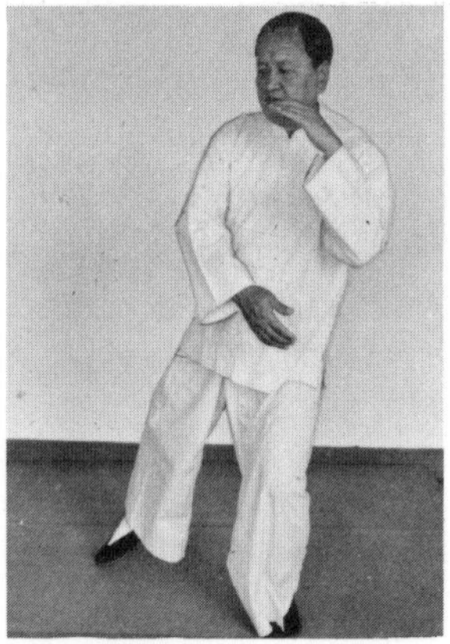

This is a 'repeat' move, one that you have learnt and practised twice before, for Positions 4 and 30. It has been described adequately and you are referred to pages 24–27 and 87–91 for a detailed description of the move.

FIG. 34-1F

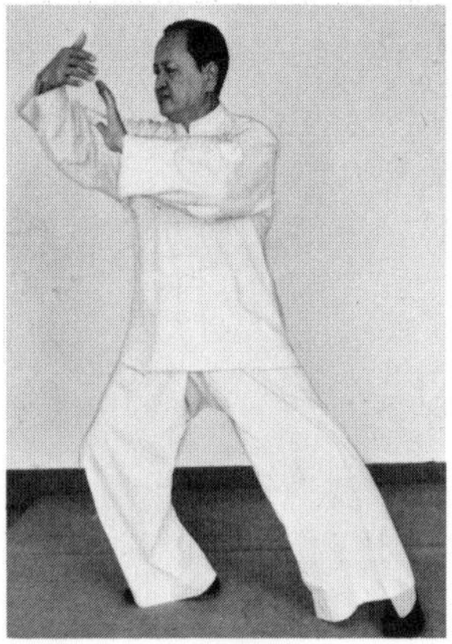

FIG. 34-2F

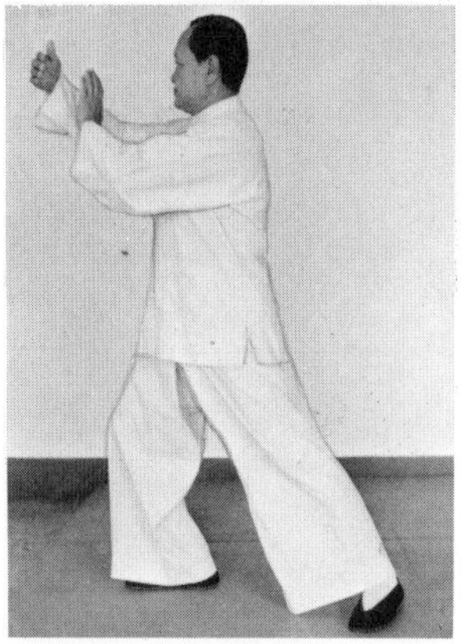

FIG. 34-3F

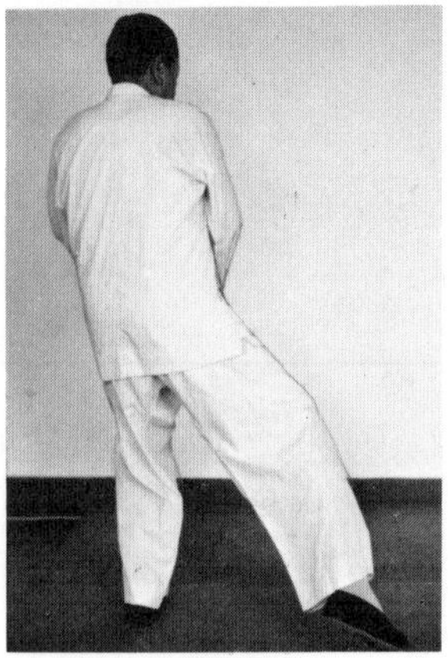

FIG. 34-1B

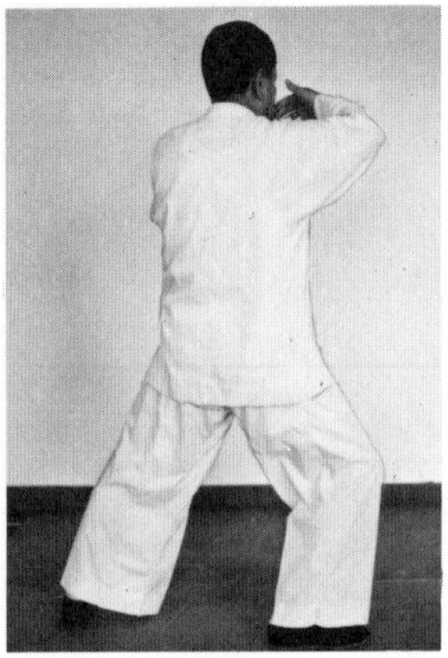

FIG. 34-2B

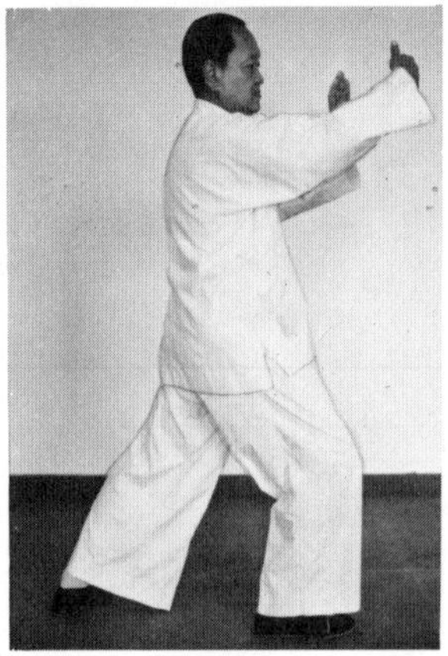

FIG. 34-3B

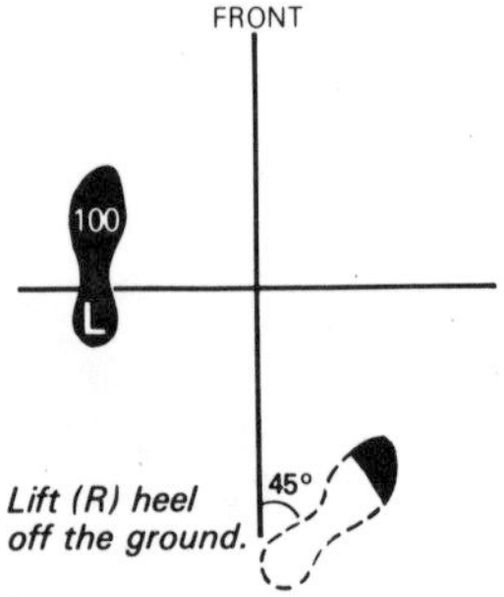

FRONT

100

L

Lift (R) heel
off the ground.

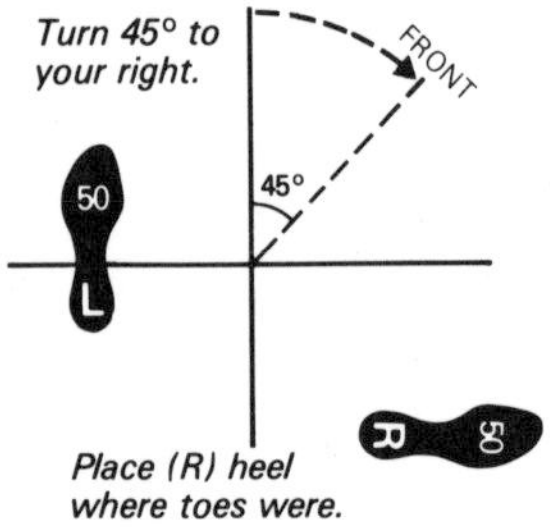

45°

*Turn 45° to
your right.*

FRONT

50

L

45°

Place (R) heel
where toes were.

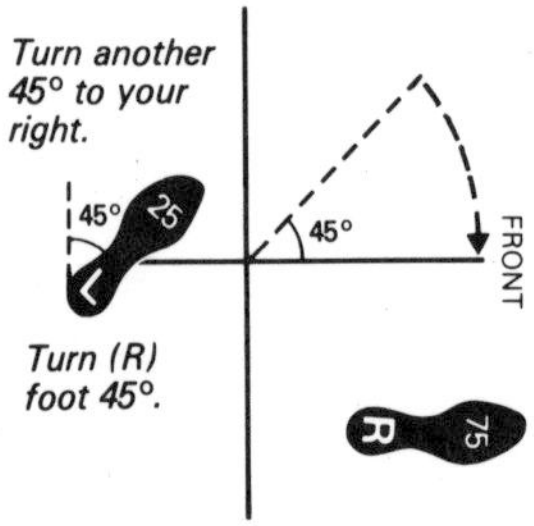

R 50

*Turn another
45° to your
right.*

45°

25

L

45°

FRONT

*Turn (R)
foot 45°.*

R 75

Shift weight to front (R) foot.

Lǎn què wěi (lí shǒu)

Grasp sparrow's tail, roll back

This second part of the move, *lí shǒu,* has also been studied in detail before. Illustrations and a description of the move are given on pages 25 and 89.

揽雀尾（攦手） *Position* 34 *(contd.)*

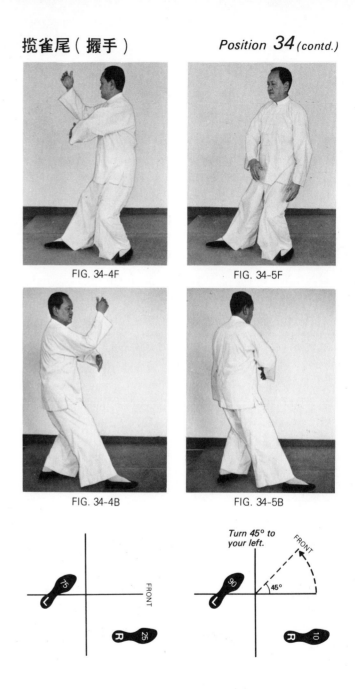

FIG. 34-4F

FIG. 34-5F

FIG. 34-4B

FIG. 34-5B

Shift weight to back (L) foot.

Position 34 (contd.) 揽雀尾（挤手）

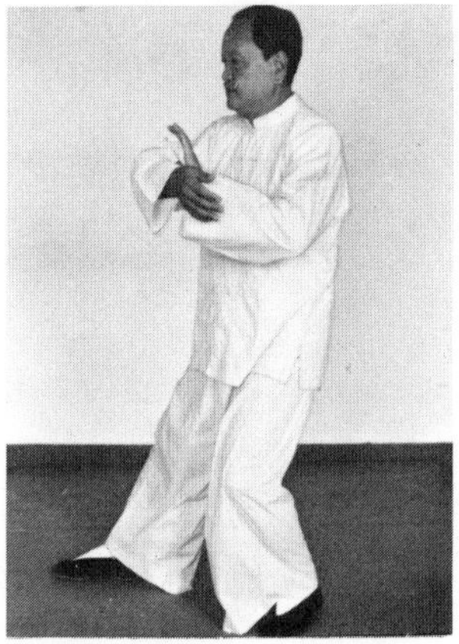

FIG. 34-6F

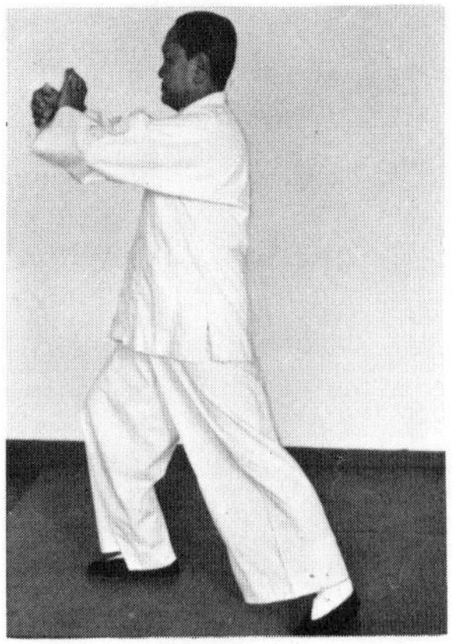

FIG. 34-7F

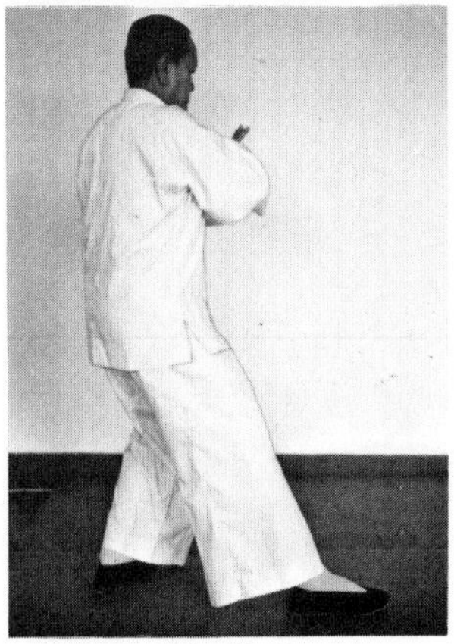

FIG. 34-6B

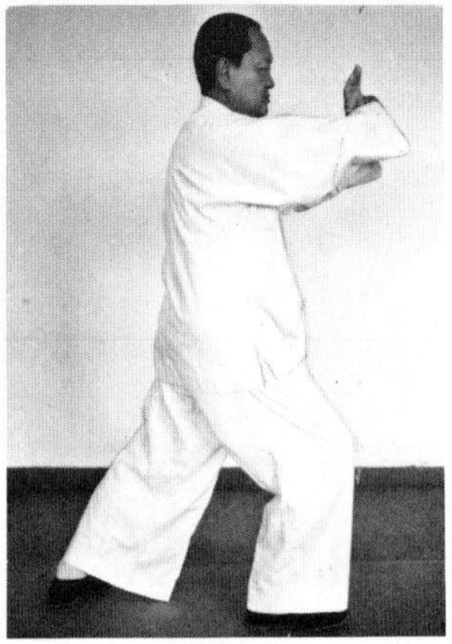

FIG. 34-7B

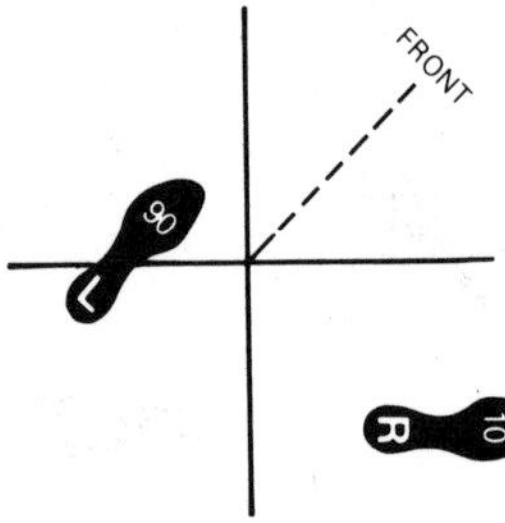
FRONT
90
L
R
10

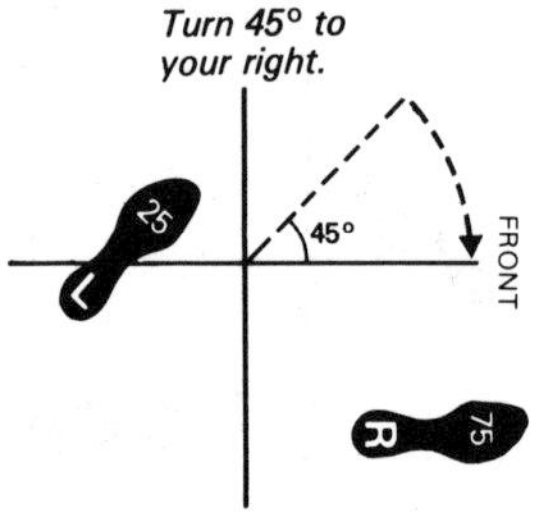
Turn 45° to your right.
25
L
45°
FRONT
R
75

Move forward. Transfer weight to front (R) foot.

Lǎn què wěi (jǐ shǒu)

Grasp sparrow's tail, press

The third part of *lǎn què wěi (jǐ shǒu)* is described on pages 26 and 90.

Lǎn què wěi (àn shǒu)

Grasp sparrow's tail, push down

Àn shǒu, the fourth part of Position 34, is described in detail on pages 27 and 91. As mentioned earlier, this complex of four moves is one of the more important parts in the exercise and hence is performed a total of four times – two were repeated at Positions 4 and 30 and the fourth, under a different name, at Position 14 *(bào hǔ guī shān).*

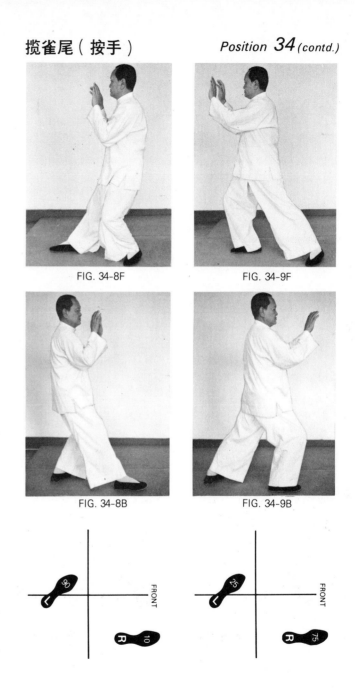

FIG. 34-8F

FIG. 34-9F

FIG. 34-8B

FIG. 34-9B

First move back onto back (L) foot.
Then move forward again onto front (R) foot.

单鞭

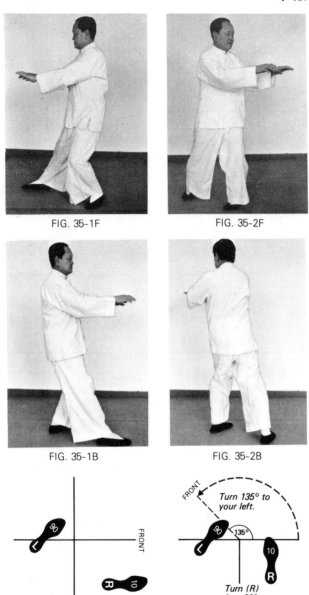

FIG. 35-1F

FIG. 35-2F

FIG. 35-1B

FIG. 35-2B

Turn 135° to
your left.

FRONT

FRONT

135°

Turn (R)
foot 90°.

Transfer weight to back (L) foot.

Dān biān
Single whip

You will probably be quite familiar with this move, having done it four times – at Positions 5 (pages 28–30), 15 (pages 50–52), 20 (pages 67–68) and 31 (pages 92–94). Please refer to the detailed description presented in earlier pages. The figures shown here are identical to those on page 28. The common errors usually relate to failure to keep weight focused on **(L) foot.** Many start shifting weight too early, before the turn is completed. Remember also never to straighten the arms completely. The elbows should always be kept slightly flexed.

单鞭

Dān biān
Single whip

The moves illustrated here are identical to those on page 29. The description of basic moves is given on that page, with the finer points presented on page 93. To recapitulate:

1 Keep your weight on **(R) foot** as you turn 135° to your right. This will become increasingly difficult as you complete the turn. The tendency is to shift your weight back to your (L) foot. Guard against this.

2 Never extend your (R) elbow completely. Always keep it slightly flexed.

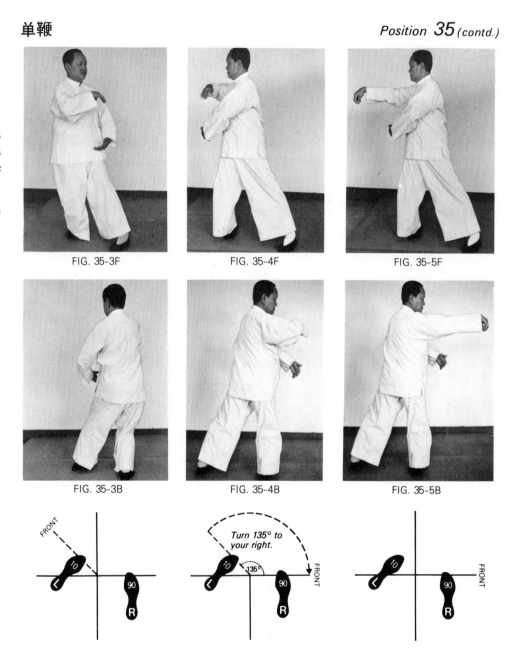

FIG. 35-3F   FIG. 35-4F   FIG. 35-5F

FIG. 35-3B   FIG. 35-4B   FIG. 35-5B

Move back. Transfer weight to (R) foot.

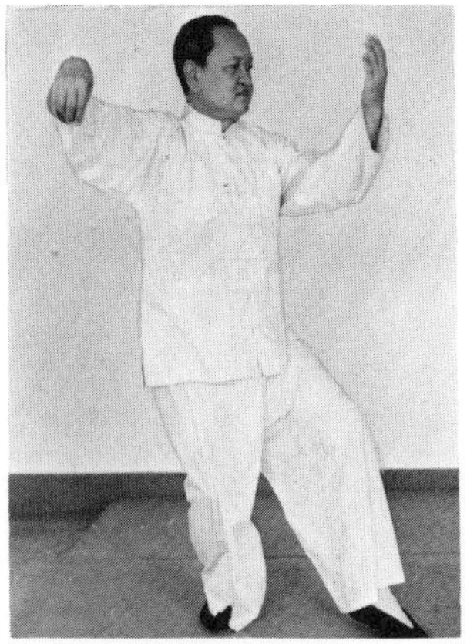

FIG. 35-6F

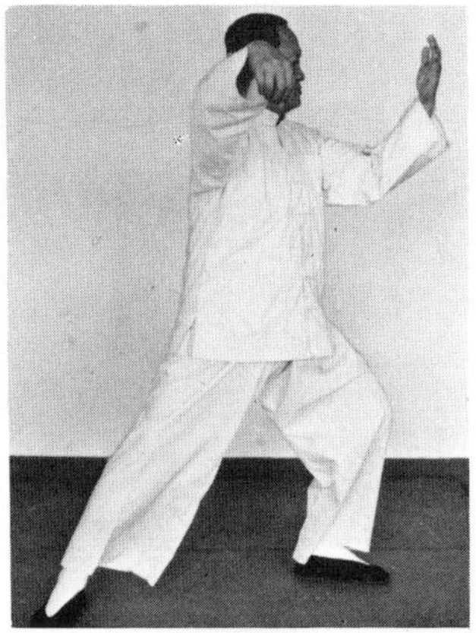

FIG. 35-7F

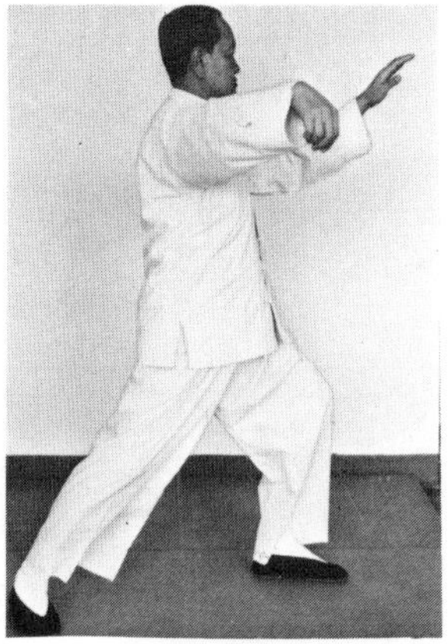

FIG. 35-8F

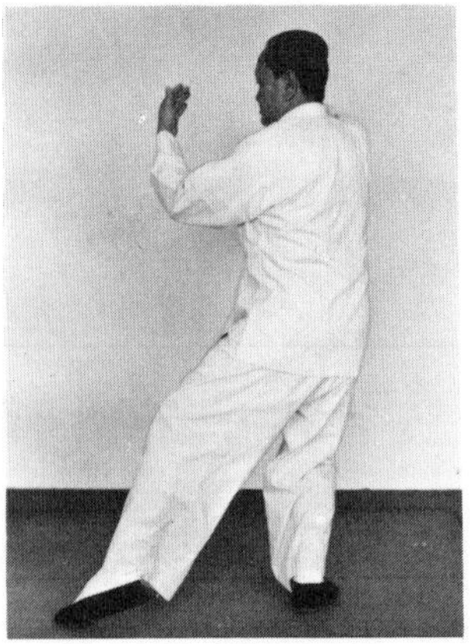

FIG. 35-6B

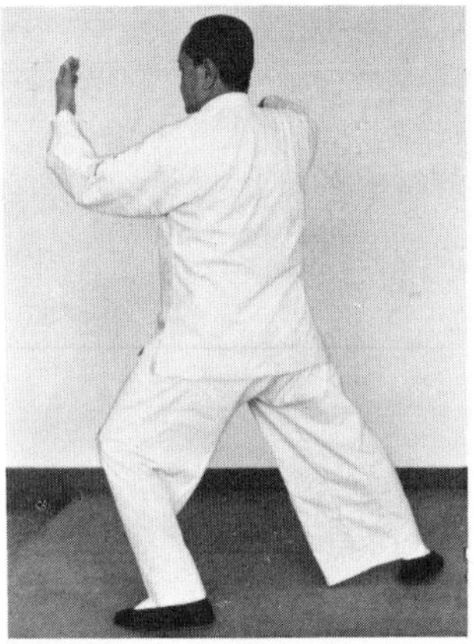

FIG. 35-7B

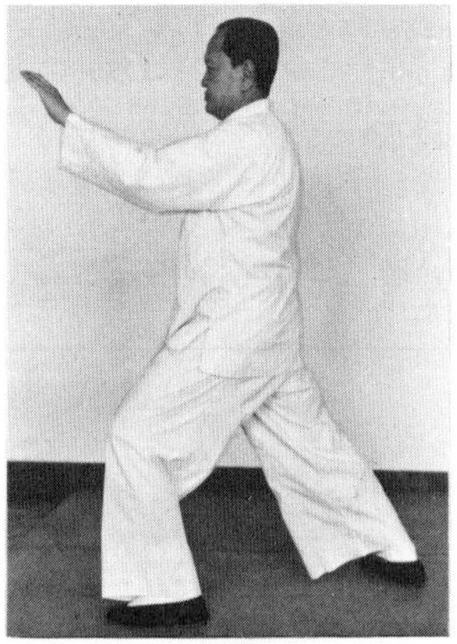

FIG. 35-8B

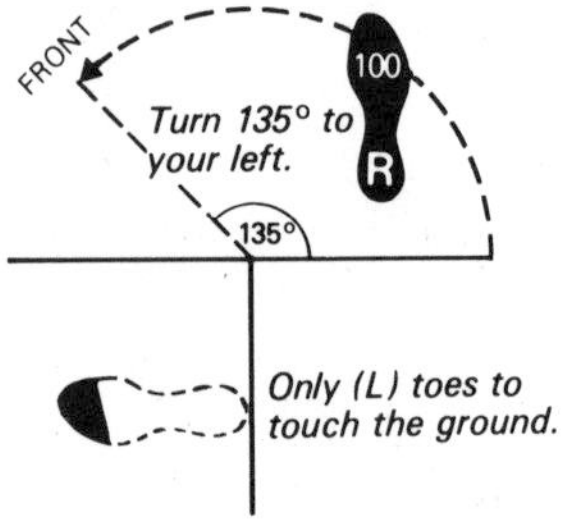

FRONT

Turn 135° to
your left.

135°

100

R

Only (L) toes to
touch the ground.

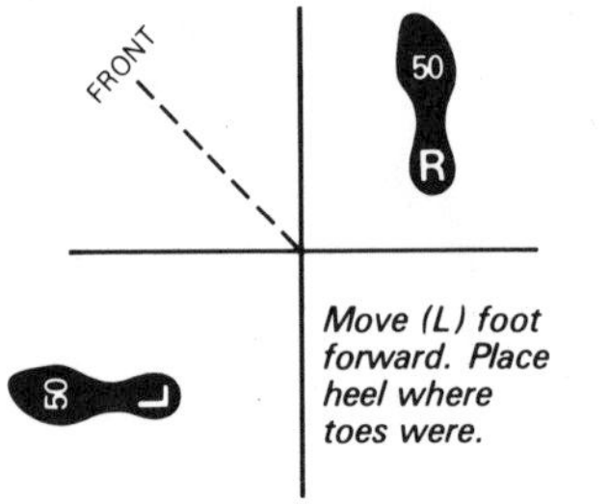

FRONT

50

R

Move (L) foot
forward. Place
heel where
toes were.

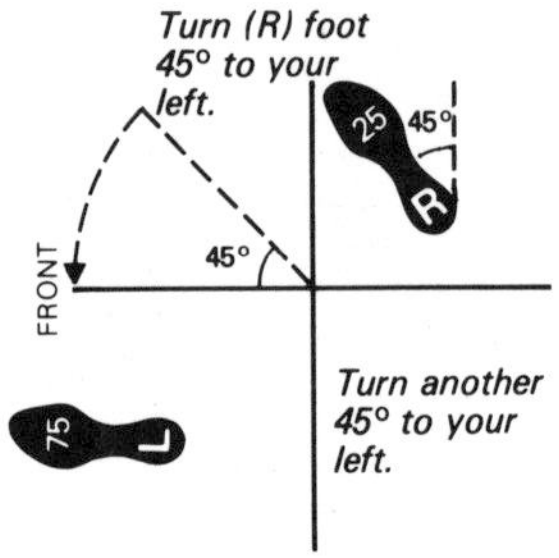

50

L

Turn (R) foot
45° to your
left.

FRONT

45°

45°

25

R

Turn another
45° to your
left.

75

L

Move forward. Shift weight to front (L) foot.

Dān biān

Single whip

The last three figures here illustrate the completion of this complex move. Remember to check with page 94 to recapitulate the finer points of this move. The very fact that you do *dān biān* five times during the course of this exercise underlines its importance to taiji. It is indeed one of the moves you would have to master thoroughly if you wish to progress in the art.

Later, when you become more proficient, this move can be used to improve your 'leg strength'. This is done by keeping absolutely still in the classic *dān biān* posture – the last move, illustrated in Fig. 35-8. Initially, you should hold yourself in this position for 5–10 seconds, gradually increasing the interval to 30 seconds and finally to 60 seconds. If there is no timepiece close at hand, time yourself by the number of breaths you take while standing still – starting from 3 and increasing gradually through 6 to 9 or 12: how quickly you progress here depends on your commitment and degree of enthusiasm.

Frequent practice helps, so hold this position for all five *dān biān* moves in this exercise. The important thing to remember is the holding period should be increased gradually. Sudden progression will not benefit you – it would cause you to begin adopting incorrect postures involuntarily or to breathe more rapidly! Also, if you do this exercise when you are fatigued or constipated, you may get giddy spells. Do not be too alarmed as you will recover very quickly if you sip a hot drink and sit down for a while. If you do arrive at this stage, it would be advisable for you to seek out a competent instructor to help you progress in your practice of the art.

Xià shì

Squatting single whip

下势

This is a 'repeat' of Position 21 (page 70). There are a few points to note when you carry out this move. First, keep weight on the **(R) foot** throughout, particularly when you squat. Many people tend to distribute their weight between both legs, especially at this juncture. This is incorrect.

Second, keep **(L) arm** fully extended and hold it close to the inner side of (L) leg. Do *not* flex (L) elbow.

Third, your **(R) arm** should also be fully extended with **(R) wrist** flexed and (R) thumb held against the second and third fingers. It helps you to maintain your balance. Finally keep **head** upright and focus **eyes** on the outstretched hand.

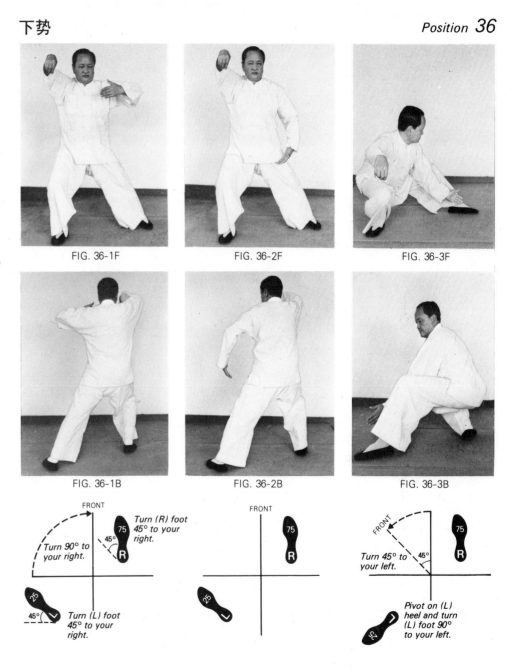

FIG. 36-1F   FIG. 36-2F   FIG. 36-3F

FIG. 36-1B   FIG. 36-2B   FIG. 36-3B

Shift weight to (R) foot.

上步七星

Shàng bù qī xīng

Step forward to seven stars

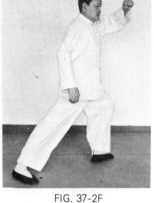

FIG. 37-1F

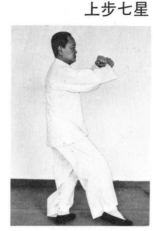

FIG. 37-2F

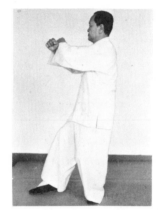

FIG. 37-3F

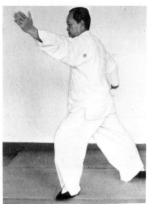

FIG. 37-1B

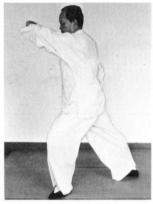

FIG. 37-2B

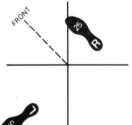

FIG. 37-3B

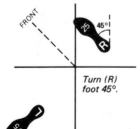

FRONT

45°

25

R

75

Turn (R) foot 45°.

FRONT

25

R

75

Turn 45° to your left.

FRONT

45°

Bring (R) foot forward. Leave only toes on the ground.

100

This is a move not previously encountered. Straighten back **(R) leg** to raise yourself till you are resting most of your weight on the front **(L) foot.** In carrying out this move turn **(R) foot** 45° to your left. As you move forward and upward, abduct **(L) shoulder** and keep **(L) elbow** extended so (L) arm is raised sideways till (L) palm is at eye level. Note that (L) arm is now directly above (L) leg with (L) elbow above (L) knee and (L) palm facing forward (Fig. 37–1). At the same time adduct **(R) shoulder** to pull (R) arm toward you. Shoulder movements should be made in conjunction with each other so that as **(L) arm** is abducted or lifted away from you, **(R) arm** is adducted or pulled toward you.

Now clench **(L) palm** into a fist and flex **(L) elbow** to pull (L) forearm toward you till it is perpendicular to the (L) upper arm. Keep **(L) shoulder** abducted so (L) fist is in front and some distance from your face (Fig. 37–2).

Finally, lift **(R) hip** and bring (R) leg forward. Allow only **(R) toes** to touch the ground at a point in front and in line with the (L) heel. All your weight must be focused on the back **(L) foot** at this point. As you move (R) leg forward, **turn** 45° to your left. Simultaneously, clench **(R) palm** into a fist, then abduct **(R) shoulder** to raise arm and cross (L) arm with (R) arm in front of you. This takes place at the wrists with the right wrist below the left (Fig. 37–3).

Transfer weight to (L) foot.

Tuì bù kuà hǔ

Step back and ride tiger

This is another new and relatively difficult move for you to master. Initially, while keeping your weight on back **(L) foot,** move **(R) leg** as far back as possible and place it down so heels of both feet form an angle of 135° between them. Keep wrists crossed in front of you (Fig. 38-1).

Maintaining this posture, with **eyes** focused on hands, rotate **both wrists** and unclench fists so the (R) palm faces you and the (L) palm faces outward (Fig. 38-2). Relax **(R) hip** and straighten (L) leg to move backward, transferring weight onto back **(R) foot.** If you bend the (R) knee as you accomplish this, you will be able to maintain the same height throughout. As you move backward, adduct **both shoulders** to allow arms to fall toward you. Keep hands crossed still so they lie in front of you with (L) wrist on top of (R) wrist (Fig. 38-3).

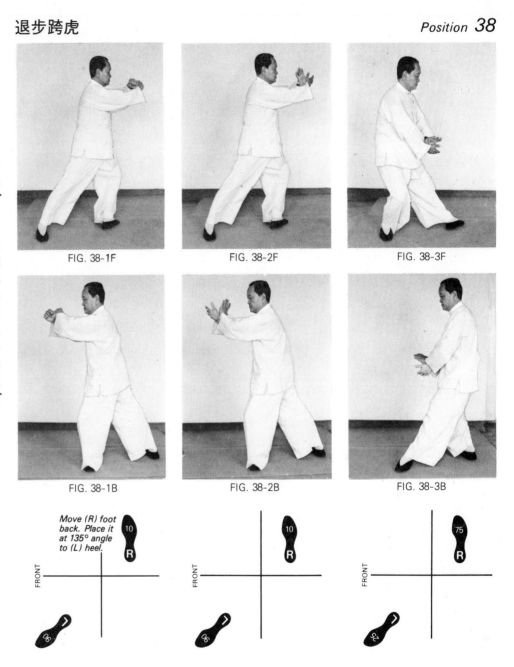

FIG. 38-1F

FIG. 38-2F

FIG. 38-3F

FIG. 38-1B

FIG. 38-2B

FIG. 38-3B

Move (R) foot back. Place it at 135° angle to (L) heel.

Transfer weight to back (R) foot.

退步跨虎

Tuì bù kuà hǔ
Step back and ride tiger

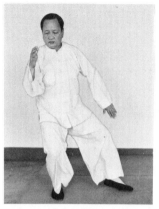
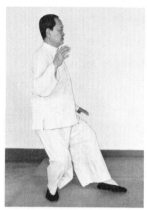
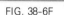

FIG. 38-4F   FIG. 38-5F   FIG. 38-6F

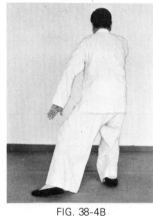
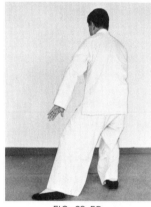
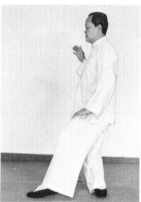

FIG. 38-4B   FIG. 38-5B   FIG. 38-6B

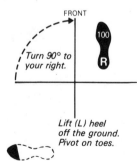
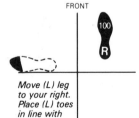
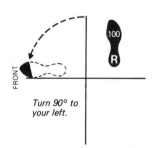

Continue the move by lifting **(L) heel** off the ground and, by pivoting on (L) toes, **turn** 90° to your right. At this point, all your weight should be on the **(R) foot.** As you execute this turn, abduct **(R) shoulder** and keep **(R) elbow** extended to raise (R) arm till it is parallel to the floor. Do not move (L) arm (Fig. 38–4).

Keeping weight on the **(R) foot,** move **(L) leg** to your right and place it such that only the toes touch the ground at a point in front and in the same line as the (R) heel. Having done this, flex **(R) elbow** then adduct **(R) shoulder** to bring (R) arm toward your body. The (R) forearm will now be upright with (R) palm facing in the same direction as your (L) foot. Do not move (L) arm (Fig. 38–5).

Finally, while keeping feet still, **turn** 90° to your left. Do not move (R) arm. Flex **(L) elbow** slightly and extend **(L) wrist** to bring (L) palm parallel to the floor. Keep weight on back **(R) foot** and allow only toes of (L) foot to touch the ground. Pull in **(L) hip** so that the hips are in line with your back (R) foot (Fig. 38–6).

FRONT

100 R

Turn 90° to your right.

Lift (L) heel off the ground. Pivot on toes.

FRONT

100 R

Move (L) leg to your right. Place (L) toes in line with (R) heel.

FRONT

100 R

Turn 90° to your left.

Keep weight on back (R) foot throughout.

Zhuǎn shēn bǎi lián
Turn body and sweep lotus with leg

This is another new move that is quite difficult to carry out. It involves turning 360° before executing a low kick. If it is not executed properly, you may well find yourself losing your balance and . falling.

First abduct and then rotate **(R) shoulder** to move (R) upper arm sideways and (R) forearm parallel to the floor with the palm facing downward. Turn **(L) wrist** so that (L) palm faces forward. Extend **(L) elbow** and subsequently adduct **(L) shoulder** to bring entire (L) arm back. Do not move any other part of your body so your weight should still be on the back **(R) leg** and only **toes** of (L) foot are in contact with the ground at this point (Fig. 39–1).

Next, while keeping both arms still, **turn** 90° to your right. Simultaneously, lift **(L) leg** and place **(L) heel** behind (R) foot. This will put you in a position where both legs are crossed, with (L) leg over the right. All your weight should still rest on the **(R) foot** (Fig. 39–2).

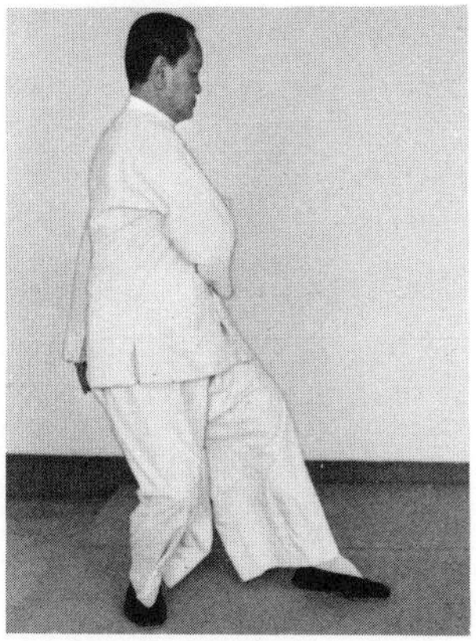

FIG. 39-1F

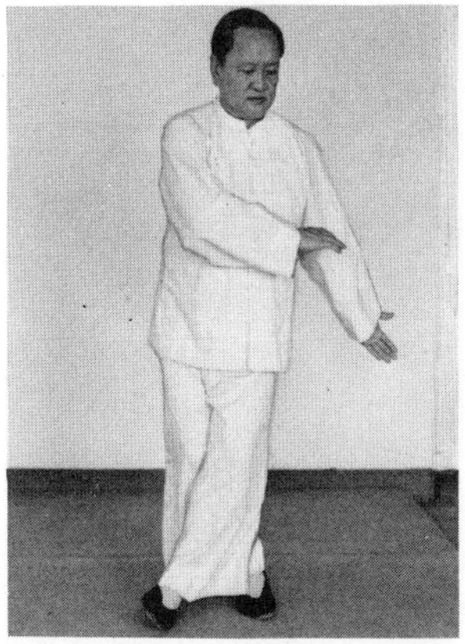

FIG. 39-2F

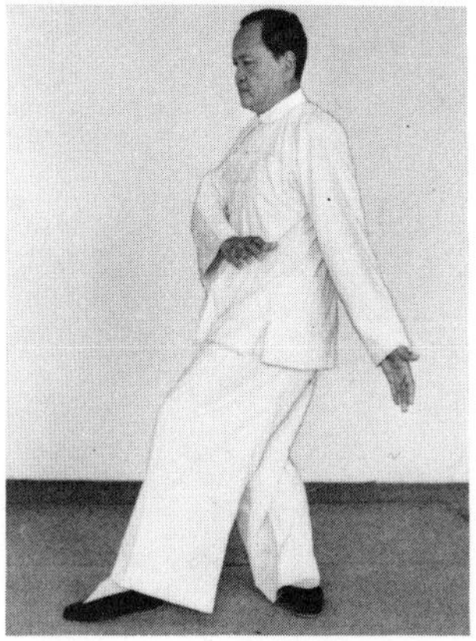

FIG. 39-1B

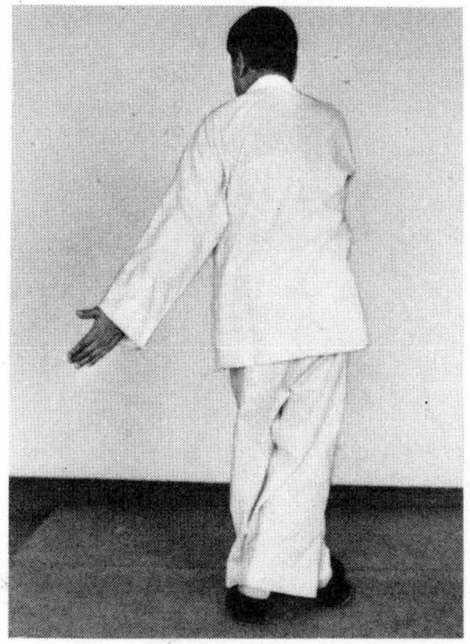

FIG. 39-2B

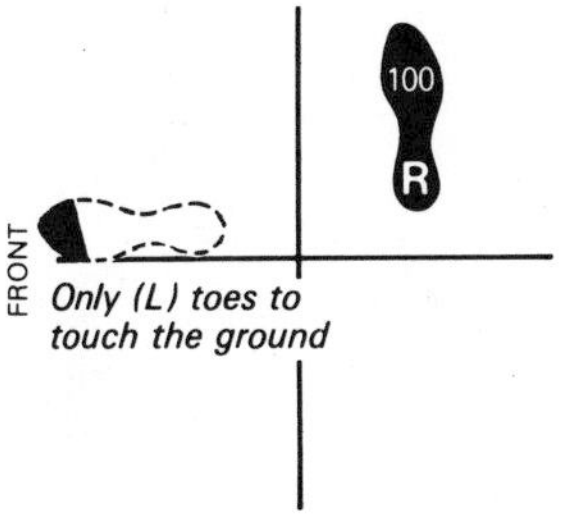

FRONT

FRONT

Only (L) toes to touch the ground

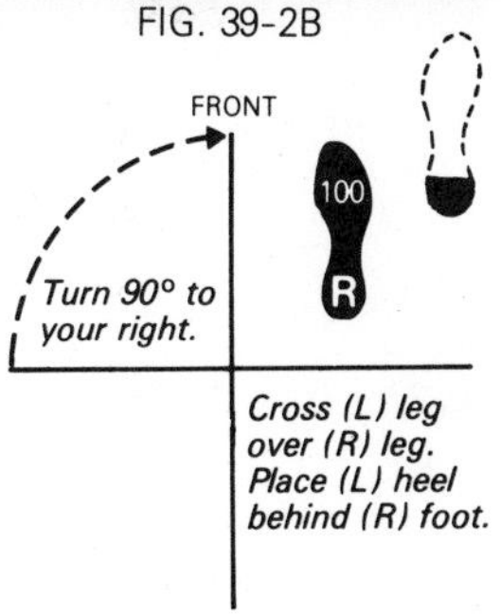

Turn 90° to your right.

Cross (L) leg over (R) leg. Place (L) heel behind (R) foot.

Keep weight on (R) foot.

转身摆莲

Zhuǎn shēn bǎi lián

Turn body and sweep lotus with leg

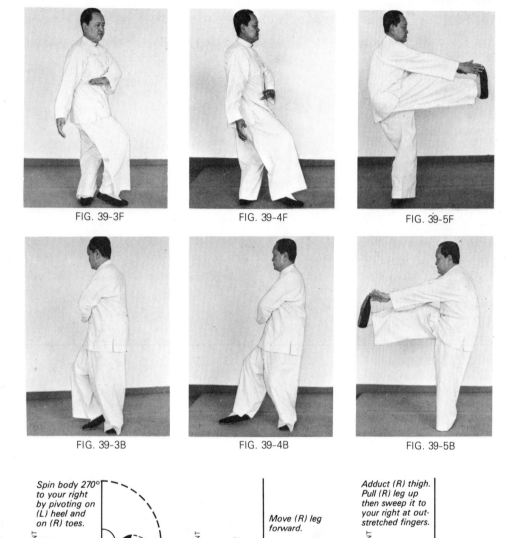

FIG. 39-3F   FIG. 39-4F   FIG. 39-5F

FIG. 39-3B   FIG. 39-4B   FIG. 39-5B

Spin body 270° to your right by pivoting on (L) heel and on (R) toes.

270°

FRONT

100

Move (R) leg forward.

FRONT

100

Adduct (R) thigh. Pull (R) leg up then sweep it to your right at outstretched fingers.

FRONT

100

Transfer weight from (R) to (L) foot as you turn.

Spin **body** 270° to your right. You would now have made a complete 360° turn. This turn should be carried out slowly by initially pivoting on **(L) heel** and **(R) toes** (for the first 90°), and then on **both** (L) and (R) heels (for the last 180°). If you use the different parts of both feet as indicated, you would be able to transfer your weight smoothly from (R) to **(L) foot** as you complete the turn. At the end of the turn you should be resting your entire weight on the **(L) foot.** Only toes of (R) foot should rest on the ground, in front of the (L) foot. Extend **(R) elbow,** then abduct **(R) shoulder** to pull (R) arm across and to the right of your body and position it behind you. Simultaneously, adduct **(L) shoulder** and then flex **(L) elbow.** This will lift (L) upper arm sideways, away from your body, while the (L) forearm is pulled across your body till it is parallel to the ground (Fig. 39-3).

When you have completed the 360° turn, move **(R) leg** forward and allow only the toes to touch the ground (Fig. 39-4). Finally, adduct **(R) hip** to lift (R) thigh parallel to the ground. Keeping the (R) leg high, adduct **(R) hip** to bring (R) leg to the left. Now flex **(R) ankle** and then sweep (R) leg across the body, from left to right. At the same time abduct **both shoulders** and then extend **both elbows** to hold the arms stretched out in front of you with **palms** facing downward. The sweep of your **(R) leg** should be directed toward outstretched fingers (Fig. 39-5).

Wān gōng shè hǔ

Bend bow and shoot tiger

This is yet another new move. When you have completed the last move, flex **(R) knee** to pull in (R) shin. Keep **(R) leg** suspended, with (R) toes pointing downward near (L) heel. At the same time adduct both **shoulders** to pull both upper arms back toward your body. Extend **(L) elbow** and allow (L) arm to hang loosely by your side. Flex **(R) elbow** to pull (R) forearm across your body with palm facing you. As you pull both arms back toward you, **turn** 45° to your left (Fig. 40–1).

Now extend **(R) knee** and place **(R) foot** as far as possible to your right and in front of the (L) foot. The heels of both feet should now describe an angle of 135° between them. Keep your weight concentrated on back **(L) foot** (Fig. 40–2).

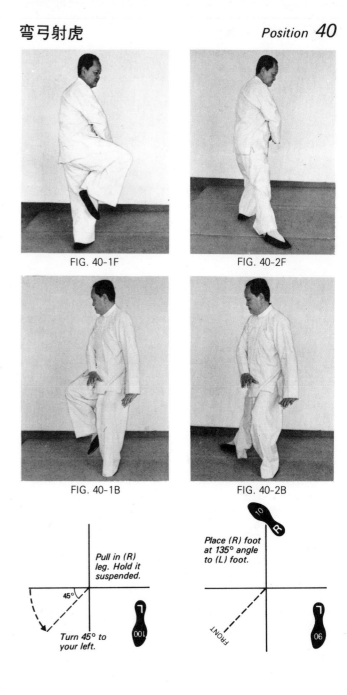

FIG. 40-1F

FIG. 40-2F

FIG. 40-1B

FIG. 40-2B

Pull in (R) leg. Hold it suspended.

45°

Turn 45° to your left.

Place (R) foot at 135° angle to (L) foot.

FRONT

Keep weight on (L) foot.

弓射虎

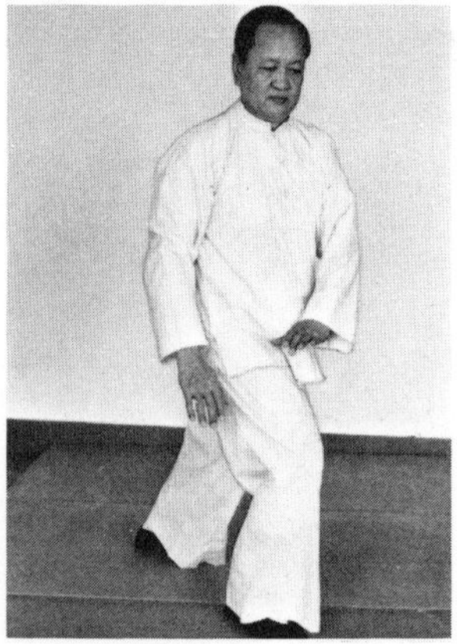

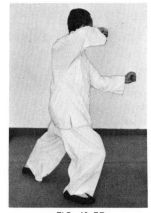

FIG. 40-3F

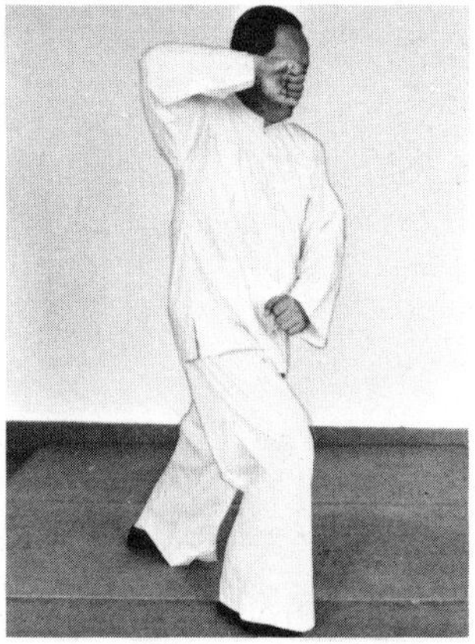

FIG. 40-4F

FIG. 40-5F

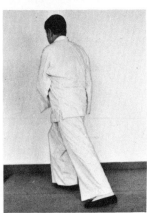

FIG. 40-3B

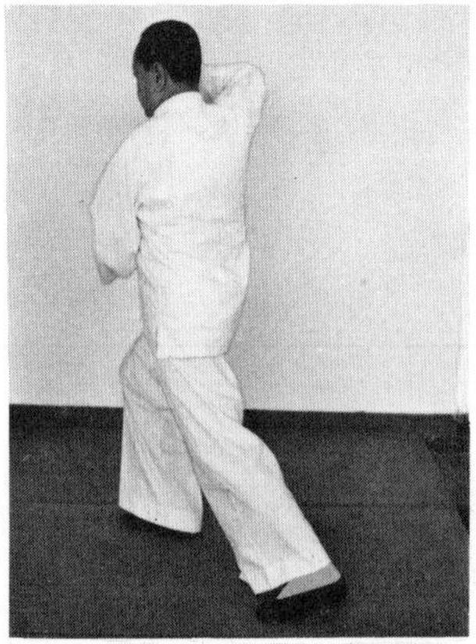

FIG. 40-4B

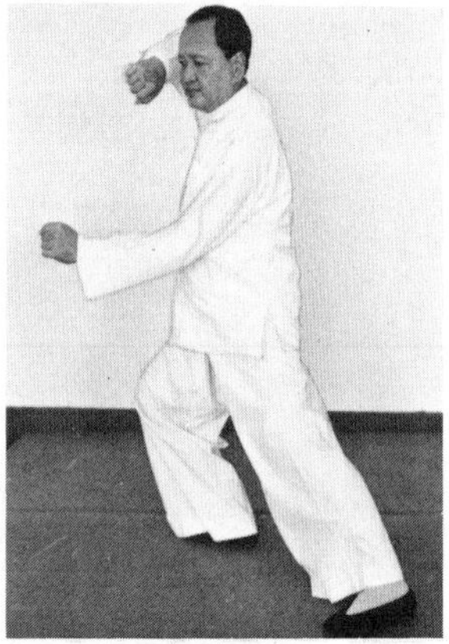

FIG. 40-5B

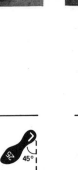
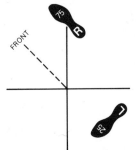

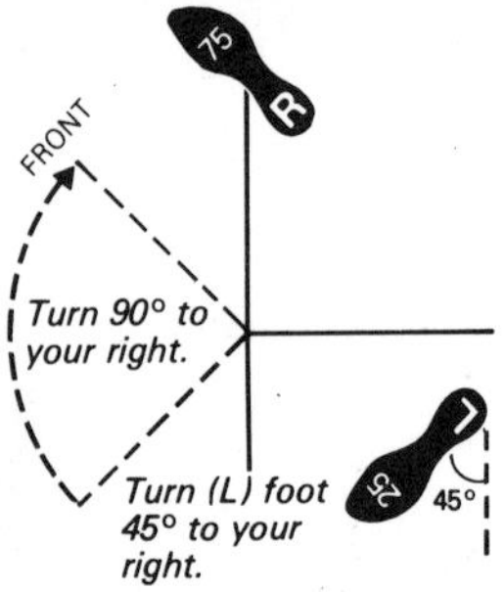

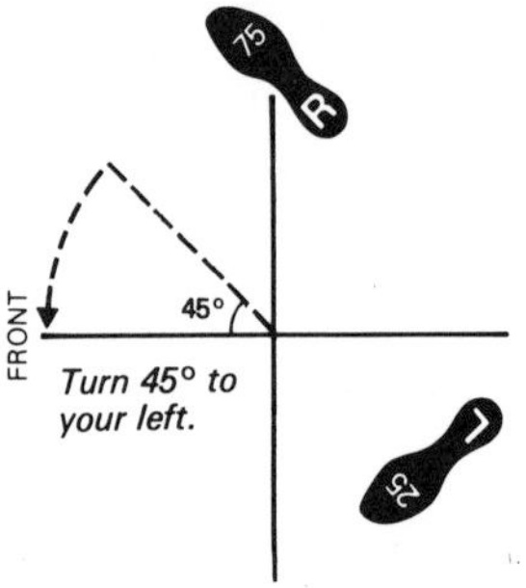

FRONT

Turn **90°** to
your right.

Turn (L) foot
45° to your
right.

FRONT

FRONT

45°

Turn **45°** to
your left.

Transfer weight to (R) foot.

Wān gōng shè hǔ

Bend bow and shoot tiger

Straighten **(L) leg** and move forward to rest most of your weight on the **(R) foot.** As you do this, **turn** 90° to your right, at the same time turning (L) foot 45° to your right. You should face the direction in which (R) foot is pointing. Keep both arms still in relation to your body with **(R) arm** beside you and (L) arm lying across your body (Fig. 40–3).

Maintaining your position, clench **(R) hand** into a fist and rotate **(R) wrist** till closed palm faces away from you. Abduct **(R) shoulder** to raise (R) upper arm laterally till (R) elbow is at shoulder level. At this point flex **(R) elbow** to bring (R) forearm toward you with knuckles of (R) fist facing you. Clench **(L) hand** into a fist (Fig. 40–4).

Finally, make a 45° **turn** to your left at the waist while keeping both feet still. Your head should turn together with your body. Keep both arms still in relation to your body and you will find that the **(L) fist** now points in the direction you face. Abduct **(L) shoulder** and keep **(L) elbow** extended so (L) forearm is thrust forward (Fig. 40–5).

Jìn bù, bān, lán chuí

Step forward, deflect downward, parry and punch

This is essentially a repeat of Position 11 on pages 39–41. The main difference lies in linking the last move of *wān gōng shè hǔ* with the first move of Position 41.

First lift (L) heel and turn **(L) foot** 45° to your left. Both heels now describe an angle of 135° between them. Simultaneously, move both elbows. First unclench **(L) fist** then flex **(L) elbow** to bring (L) palm beside (R) elbow. At the same time extend **(R) elbow** to lift (R) fist away from you (Fig. 41-1).

Now straighten front **(R) leg** to move back and transfer weight onto back **(L) foot**. At the same time **turn** 45° to your left and bring both arms down in the following fashion.

Adduct **(R) shoulder** to bring (R) arm toward you, keeping **(R) elbow** extended so (R) arm moves as one unit till (R) fist lies in front of you. At the same time adduct **(L) shoulder** then extend **(L) elbow** to bring entire (L) arm down till it lies beside you with (L) palm facing downward. The movement of the (L) arm should be carried out in stages – first adduct (L) shoulder to bring (L) upper arm down and only when it is in position should you extend your elbow. The principle involved here is that only one joint in a limb should be moved at any one time (Fig. 41-2).

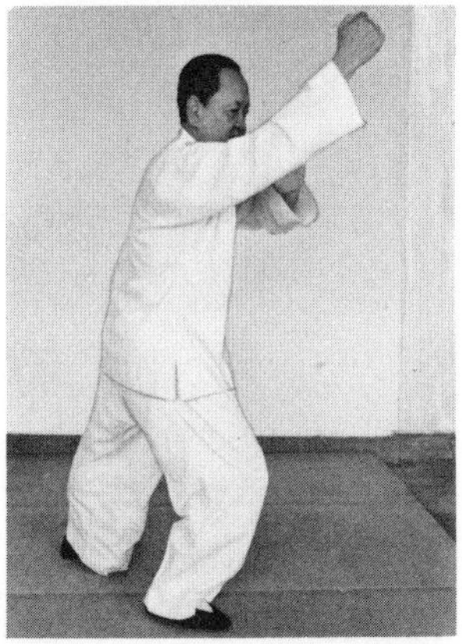

FIG. 41-1F

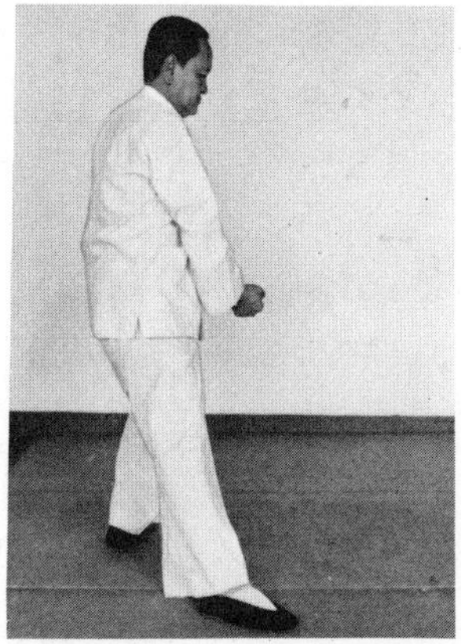

FIG. 41-2F

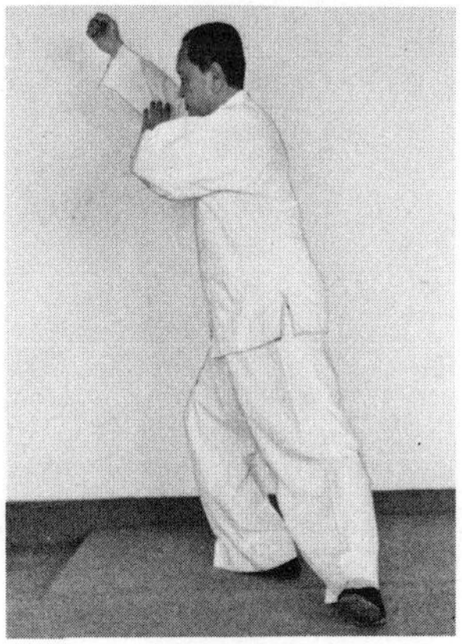

FIG. 41-1B

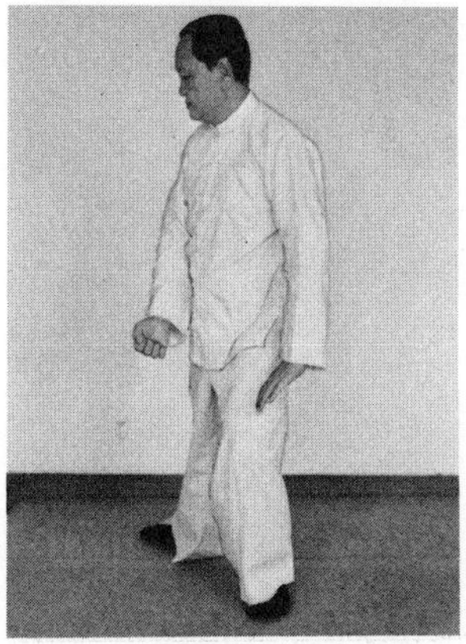

FIG. 41-2B

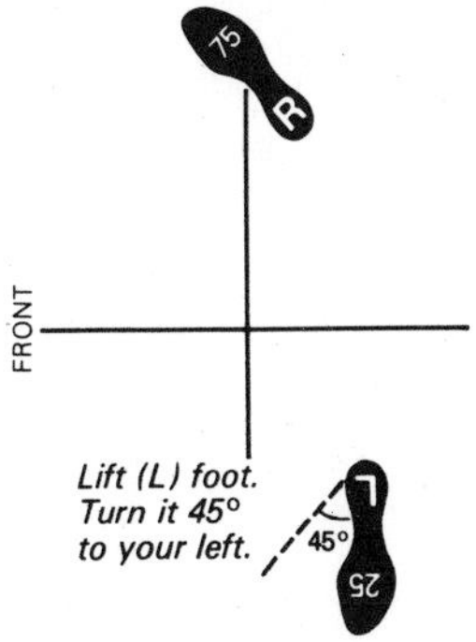

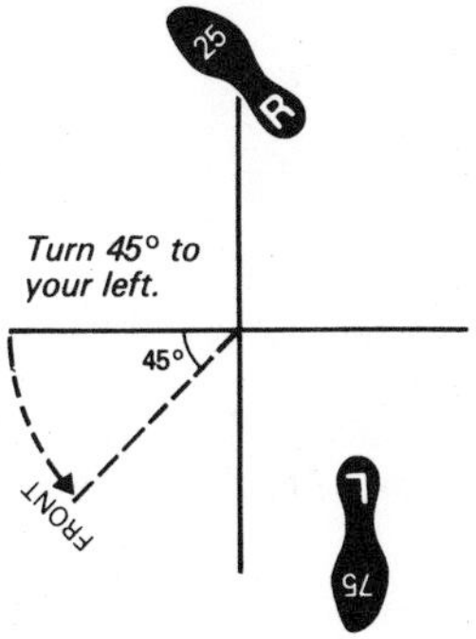

FRONT

Lift (L) foot.
Turn it 45°
to your left.

45°

Turn 45° to
your left.

45°

FRONT

Transfer weight to back (L) foot.

进步搬拦捶

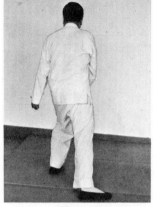

FIG. 41-3F

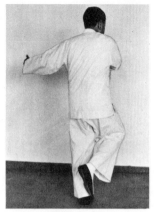

FIG. 41-4F

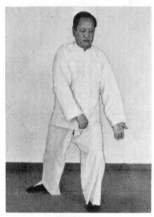

FIG. 41-3B

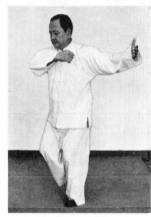

FIG. 41-4B

Jìn bù, bān, lán chuí

Step forward, deflect downward, parry and punch

Keeping weight on the **(L) foot, turn** another 45° to your left. Synchronise this turn of your body with a similar rotation of the **(R) foot** so feet are now perpendicular to each other. Keep both hands still but rotate **(L) wrist** so open (L) palm now faces forward, in the same direction as your body. Keep **(R) hand** clenched (Fig. 41–3).

The next sequence of moves is identical to that described for Position 11 on pages 39–41. First lift **(R) foot,** bring it forward and hold it suspended near (L) heel. As you move forward **turn** 45° to your right and simultaneously lift both arms. Keeping (L) elbow extended, abduct **(L) shoulder** to raise entire (L) arm until it is parallel to the ground. At the same time abduct **(R) shoulder** till (R) arm is parallel to the ground, then flex **(R) elbow** to bring (R) fist to the centre of your chest (Fig. 41–4).

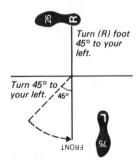

Turn (R) foot 45° to your left.

Turn 45° to your left. / 45°

FRONT 75

Lift (R) foot off the ground. Hold it suspended near (L) heel.

Turn back 45°. 45°

FRONT 100

Keep weight on (L) foot.

Jìn bù, bān, lán chuí

*Step forward, deflect downward,
parry and punch*

Continue by extending (R) **knee** to place
(R) heel on the ground in front of and perpendicular to (L) heel. Your weight should
still be concentrated on the (L) **foot**. As
you step out move both elbows simultaneously. Flex the (L) **elbow** to bring open
(L) palm beside your ear and extend (R)
elbow to lift (R) forearm to an almost upright position (Fig. 41–5).

Turn (R) **foot** 90° to the right and
straighten back (L) leg by lifting (L) **heel**
off the ground. This will propel you forward onto the front (R) **foot** which should
now carry entire weight. As you execute
this move, **turn** 90° to your right. Keeping
(L) elbow flexed, abduct (L) **shoulder** to
bring (L) arm forward. At the same time
adduct (R) **shoulder** to allow (R) arm to
fall to your side (Fig. 41–6).

Now, step forward and place (L) **foot** in
front of and perpendicular to the (R) heel.
Keep weight focused on (R) foot and arms
still (Fig. 41–7). Finally, straighten back
(R) **leg** and move forward, shifting weight
onto front (L) foot. Turn **body** and (R)
foot 45° to your left and at the same time
flex (L) **elbow** to bring (L) forearm down
across your body and parallel to the ground.
Simultaneously, abduct (R) **shoulder** and,
keeping (R) **elbow** partially extended,
execute a forward punch with (R) forearm
parallel and (R) knuckles perpendicular to
the ground (Fig. 41–8). Note that (L) hand
is next to (R) elbow.

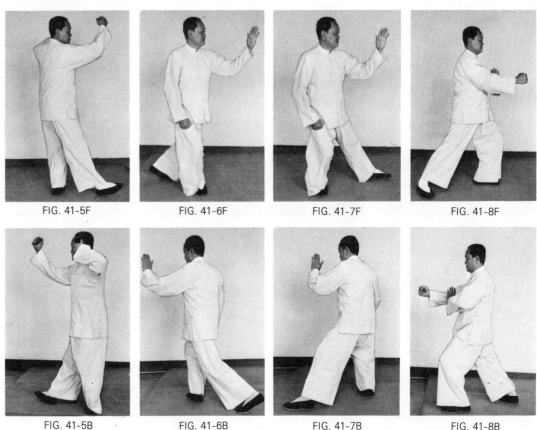

FIG. 41–5F   FIG. 41–6F   FIG. 41–7F   FIG. 41–8F

FIG. 41–5B   FIG. 41–6B   FIG. 41–7B   FIG. 41–8B

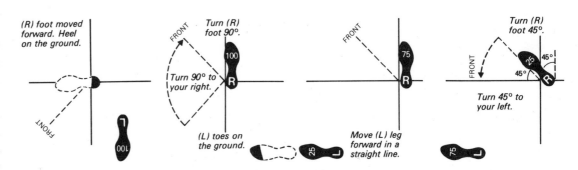

*Step forward. Transfer weight to (R) foot. Then
move forward to shift weight to front (L) foot.*

如封似闭

Rú fēng sì bì

Withdraw and push

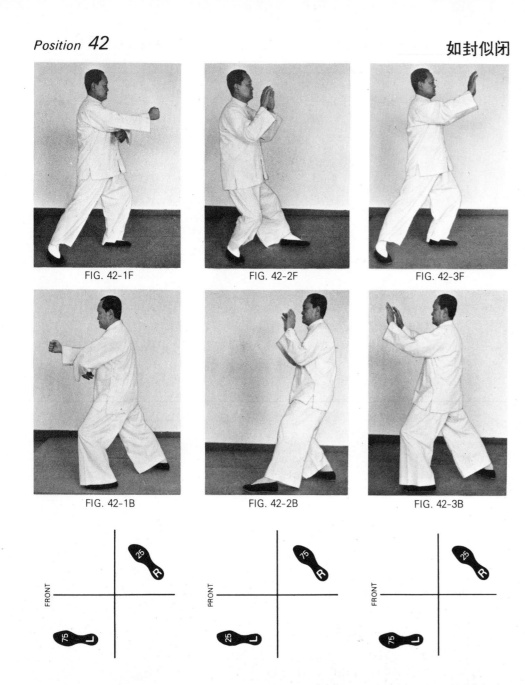

FIG. 42-1F

FIG. 42-2F

FIG. 42-3F

FIG. 42-1B

FIG. 42-2B

FIG. 42-3B

This is a repeat of Position 12. Details of the moves involved are presented on page 42 and will not be repeated here.

A few points, however, bear elaboration. As you move back onto your **(R) foot,** allow both arms to sink completely to your side (Fig. 42-2). Stretch shoulders as much as possible by allowing elbows to sink downward. Do not move forward until elbows are in place. Avoid pulling elbows behind or allowing them to settle in front of your body.

Another point worth remembering is that when you thrust forward (Fig. 42-3), the power of the thrust should be generated from your back (R) leg and not from your arms. Keep both forearms relaxed and stretch shoulders by pushing at your elbows.

The meaning of *rú fēng sì bì* – 'apparent closure' – becomes clear as this move feigns a quick withdrawal to allow for a stronger and more powerful attack.

Move back and then forward to shift weight to front (L) foot.

Shí zì shǒu

Cross hands

This is another position studied earlier (Position 13 on pages 43–44). Again we intend only to highlight a few points here.

The first part involves moving back onto your **(R) leg** (Fig. 43–1), **turning** 90° to your right and abducting both **shoulders** to raise upper arms laterally until they are parallel to the ground. As your **elbows** remain flexed, both forearms remain in a near upright position with the palms facing outward or away from your body. There are two important points to note here:

1 The movement of your arms is the result of the abduction of your shoulders – and not your elbows. It should result in your shoulders being stretched.
2 The turn of your body results in the transfer of your weight onto your front **(R) foot** (Fig. 43–2).

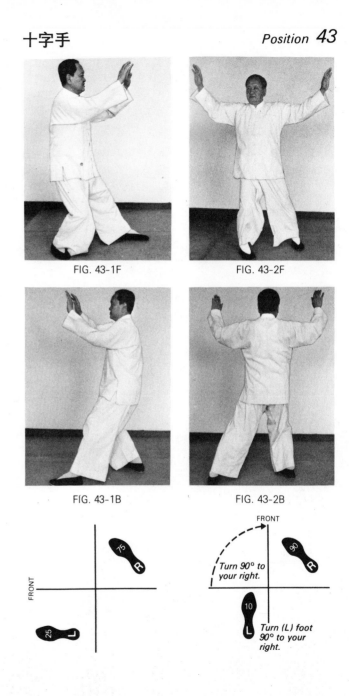

FIG. 43-1F

FIG. 43-2F

FIG. 43-1B

FIG. 43-2B

Move back. Transfer weight to (R) foot.

十字手

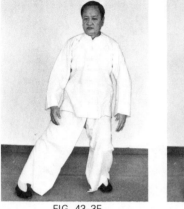

FIG. 43-3F

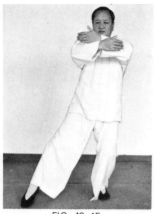

FIG. 43-4F

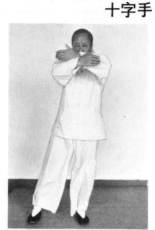

FIG. 43-5F

Shí zì shǒu
Cross hands

The remaining three parts of *shí zì shǒu* are similar to those of Position 13 described on page 44.

It involves moving back, shifting weight onto the **(L) foot** while simultaneously adducting both **shoulders** to allow arms to fall to your sides (Fig. 43-3).

Then, while you raise your **(R) heel** off the ground, abduct **shoulders** to raise arms forward till they are parallel to the ground. Then flex **elbows** to cross forearms in front of you with (R) forearm on the outside of the left. Both **palms** should be open and facing you (Fig. 43-4).

Finally, maintaining the position of your arms, draw **(R) foot** back and place it in line with the (L) foot. Weight should still be concentrated on the **(L) foot** (Fig. 43-5).

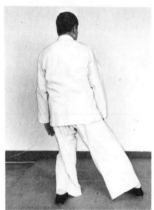

FIG. 43-3B

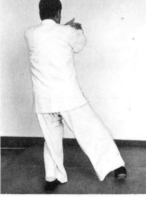

FIG. 43-4B

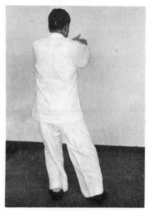

FIG. 43-5B

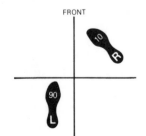

FRONT

90
L

10
R

Shift weight to (L) foot.

FRONT

100
L

Lift (R) heel off the ground.

FRONT

Bring (R) foot back.

90
L

10
R

Hé tài jí

Conclusion

This is the last movement of the exercise. Only in this and the first position of the exercise do you maintain equal distribution of weight on both **feet** throughout the move.

First relax **(R) hip** and, by straightening (L) leg slightly, ensure that your weight is equally distributed on both feet. As you carry this out adduct both **shoulders** to pull forearms apart until they are upright and elbows point downward. Now rotate wrists so palms point forward (Fig. 44–1).

Finally, adduct **shoulders** again to bring upper arms to either side of your body, then extend **elbows** to allow forearms to fall to your sides (Fig. 44–2). This completes the entire exercise.

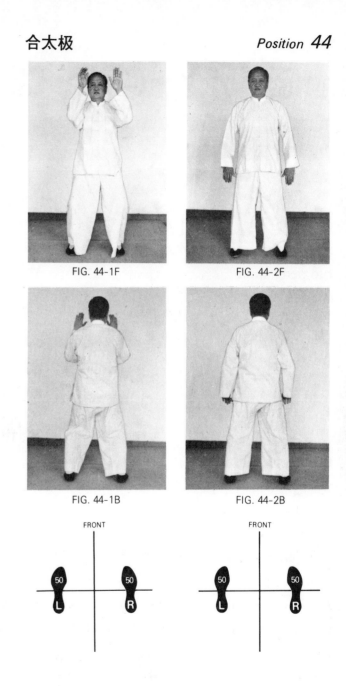

FIG. 44-1F

FIG. 44-2F

FIG. 44-1B

FIG. 44-2B

FRONT   FRONT

Keep weight evenly distributed on both feet.

Summary of Yang's Tai Chi

Chapter One 第一节

Position	Name		Pages	Repeated in Positions
1	yù bèi shì	预备式	20	
2	tài jí qǐ shì	太极起势	21–22	
3	zuǒ péng shǒu	左棚手	23	33
4	lǎn què wěi	揽雀尾		30, 34
	péng shǒu	棚手	24	
	lí shǒu	摵手	25	
	jí shǒu	挤手	26	
	àn shǒu	按手	27	
5	dān biān	单鞭	28–30	15, 20, 31, 35
6	tí shǒu	提手		
	shàng shì	上势	31	
	fù kào	附靠	32	
7	bái hè liàng chì	白鹤亮翅	33	
8	zuǒ lǒu xī aǒ bù	左搂膝拗步	34–35	10, 27
9	shǒu huī pí pa	手挥琵琶	36	
10	zuǒ lǒu xī aǒ bù	左搂膝拗步	37–38	8, 27
11	jìn bù, bān, lán chuí	进步搬拦捶	39–41	41
12	rú fēng sì bì	如封似闭	42	42
13	shí zì shǒu	十字手	43–44	43

Chapter Two 第二节

Position	Name		Pages	Repeated in Positions
14	bào hǔ guī shān	抱虎归山	46–49	
15	xié dān biān	斜单鞭	50–52	5, 20, 31, 35
16	zhǒu dǐ kàn chuí	肘底看捶	53–55	
17	dào niǎn hóu	倒撵猴	56–59	
18	xié fēi shì	斜飞势	60–61	
19	yún shǒu	云手	62–66	
20	dān biān	单鞭	67–68	5, 15, 31, 35

Final Word

Having invested so much time and effort in learning tai chi, you should now proceed to practise it on a regular basis. To do this you will need:

A PLACE
- that is quiet,
- that is about 15 metres square,
- that is flat with no stones or any other projections on the floor,
- that is preferably enclosed and well ventilated.

CLOTHING
- flat-soled shoes,
- loose and baggy pants,
- a cotton shirt – long-sleeved preferably if you are going to practise in the open.

TIME
- a minimum of ten minutes daily, if possible in the morning, to carry out one set of the exercise (44 moves) and three to five relaxation exercises,
- if you feel up to it, 30 minutes to carry out three sets of the exercise daily.

You will find (if you have maintained a daily practice schedule) that you will feel revitalised and full of energy within a short time. It is really simple – so little fuss and bother. All that is required is TEN MINUTES OF YOUR TIME DAILY!

The only real difficulty is the maintenance of a regular daily schedule. It is ever so easy to find excuses to miss just that one daily session – there will be all kinds of good, valid reasons too. Remember, however, that there is always time, if you really wish to become proficient, particularly since it is only ten minutes! A short time to develop and maintain a healthy lifestyle.

Master Chia Siew Pang

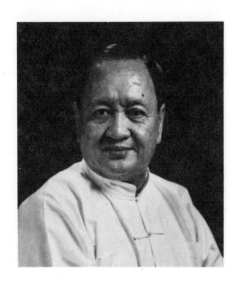

Master Chia first learnt tai chi in 1933 from Master Li Yue in Kwangtung. In 1936 he studied the art under Master Cheng Mun-ch'ng. Both his masters were students of Master Yang Cheng-fu who was largely responsible for the propagation and popularisation of Yang's tai chi.

Master Chia began teaching Yang's tai chi in Singapore in 1948, his first classes being held at the premises of the Chin Woo Association. He has been teaching tai chi ever since in Singapore, and occasionally in places as far away as Padua, Rome and London. For the last thirty years, Master Chia has had many students, including foreign dignitaries, mainly at the Tai Chi Centre in Singapore, though he has on request conducted classes at various ministries and at a community centre.

Not as generally well-known as his tai chi skills is the fact that Master Chia is an accomplished physician trained in administering traditional Chinese medicine. This is because he has given up his practice to concentrate on teaching tai chi. His interests, apart from tai chi, include Chinese art, particularly Chinese calligraphy.

Dr Goh Ewe Hock

Dr Goh is a medical practitioner, trained in western medicine and specialising in community medicine. His first involvement with Chinese martial arts took place in Singapore when, still a medical student, he studied *ngoh chor* under Mr Lim Ee Chiok. In 1972, he studied Yang's tai chi under Master Chia Siew Pang and today he practises only tai chi chuan.

Dr Goh lives in Sydney where he conducts small private classes in Yang's tai chi.

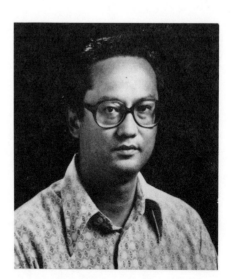